What should be done for the baby at home?

Should mental and physical developmental problems be expected in the future?

and many more.

you are expecting a new baby, or if the ew baby in your life was born a bit too arly, look to *The Littlest Baby* for the medical and practical guidance you need.

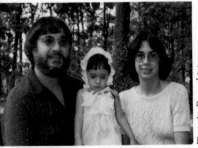

Photo by Roger Lintner

Fred, Falecia, & Faye Pfister

Fred R. Pfister is an associate professor of English at The School of the Ozarks at Pt. Lookout in Missouri.

Bernard Griesemer, M.D., is a practicing pediatrician in Springfield, Missouri. He was Falecia's doctor at the time of her birth and devotes much of his practice to premature babies.

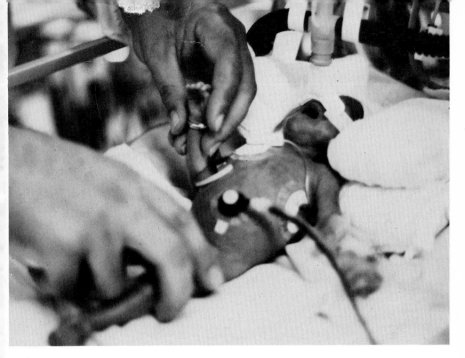

Falecia, even at a month, could wear her
father's wedding ring as a too-large bracelet.

Preemies, no matter how small,
feel pain and respond to their environment,
as Falecia seems to here.

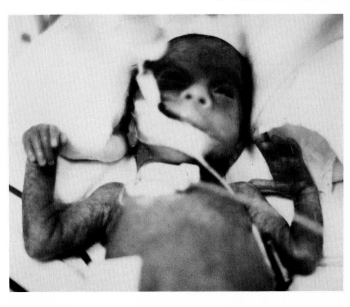

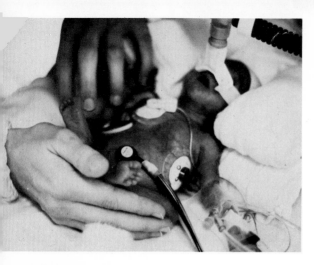

Falecia, in an open "hot crib,"
is fondled by her mother.

Falecia is held by her mother for the
first time, but still wears an oxygen mask.

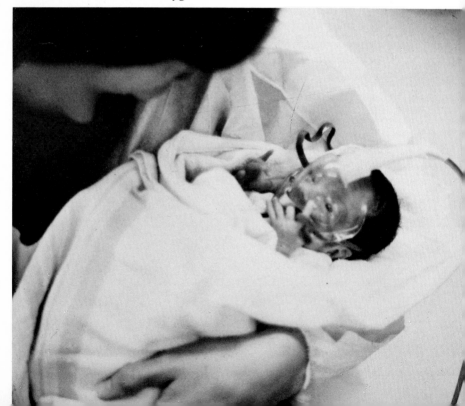

Covered by heart and oxygen monitor patches
and a silver dollar to show scale, Falecia finally
graduated to an oxyhood 6½ weeks after birth.

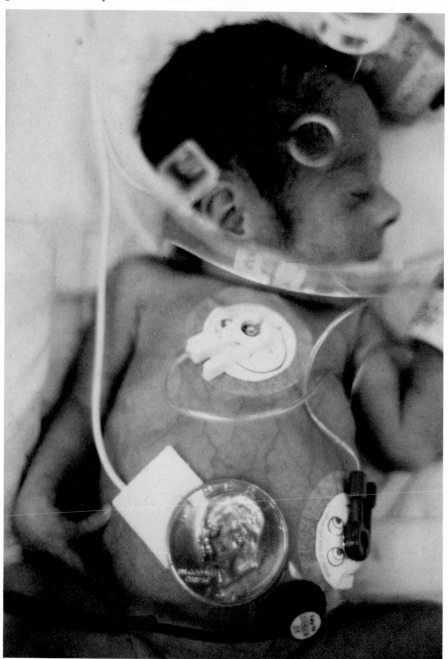

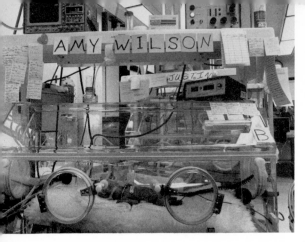

Surrounded by doctors' notes,
nurses' memos,
and the tubes
and wires of technology,
a "kilogram kid"
fights for life.
(*Photo by Beverly Robb*)

Dwarfed by her name
on the incubator, a preemie
struggles for life in
an alien atmosphere.
(*Photo by Beverly Robb*)

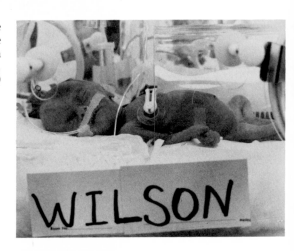

Falecia, even at 5 months,
is dwarfed by her
menagerie of stuffed animals.

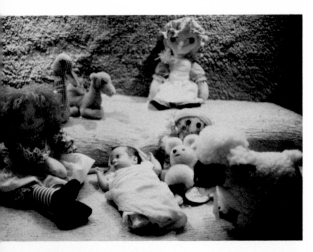

THE LITTLEST BABY

Fred Pfister is an associate professor of English at The School of the Ozarks in Point Lookout, Missouri.

Bernard Griesemer, M.D., is a practicing pediatrician in Springfield, Missouri. He was Falecia's doctor at the time of her birth, and he devotes much of his practice to premature babies.

A Handbook for Parents
of Premature Children

THE
LITTLEST
BABY

FRED R. PFISTER
BERNARD GRIESEMER, M.D.

A SPECTRUM BOOK

Prentice-Hall, Inc., Englewood Cliffs, New Jersey 07632

Library of Congress Cataloging in Publication Data

Pfister, Fred.
 The littlest baby.

 "A Spectrum Book."
Includes index.
 1. Infants (Premature)   I. Griesemer, Bernard.
II. Title.
RJ250.P48 1983   618.92'011   82-25539
ISBN 0-13-537795-1
ISBN 0-13-537787-0 (pbk.)

This book is available at a special discount when ordered in
bulk quantities. Contact Prentice-Hall, Inc., General
Publishing Division, Special Sales, Englewood Cliffs, N.J. 07632

1 2 3 4 5 6 7 8 9 10

ISBN 0-13-537795-1

ISBN 0-13-537787-0 {PBK.}

Editorial/production supervision by Kimberly Mazur
Cover design by Hal Siegel
Insert layout by Maria Carella
Manufacturing buyer: Doreen Cavallo

The findings and recommendations of the Ad Hoc Task Force of
the American Academy of Pediatrics concerning circumcision is
reprinted from *Pediatrics*, vol. 56, 4, pp. 610–11. Copyright
American Academy of Pediatrics 1975.

Prentice-Hall International, Inc., London
Prentice-Hall of Australia Pty. Limited, Sydney
Prentice-Hall Canada Inc., Toronto
Prentice-Hall of India Private Limited, New Delhi
Prentice-Hall of Japan, Inc., Tokyo
Prentice-Hall of Southeast Asia Pte. Ltd., Singapore
Whitehall Books Limited, Wellington, New Zealand
Editora Prentice-Hall do Brasil Ltda., Rio de Janeiro

For Faye, and all other mothers, past and future.

One good mother is worth a hundred school masters.

GEORGE HERBERT

An ounce of mother is worth a pound of clergy.

Spanish proverb

CONTENTS

PREFACE

Falecia is just one of many of Nature's littlest miracles. Falecia was a premature baby, one of the hundreds born every day in the United States. Her first three months in this world and the story behind them were the motivating factors for this book.

Falecia's story is dramatic only in the sense that every story of a baby requiring care in an intensive care nursery is dramatic, and every parent has the same fears and frustrations as Falecia's parents. Certainly babies smaller than Falecia have survived, and there are babies who have had more serious problems. Falecia's story may, therefore, not even be typical, but there is no such thing as a "typical" premature baby. Every one is an individual.

Falecia's story is different from the others because she was the prime mover for something for which there was a great need. Previously, there was only scattered information—insufficient hospital pamphlets and magazine articles—for the parents of premature babies. There was a wealth of specialized information for pediatricians and neonatologists. But there was nothing to explain to parents in plain and simple language what they and their baby in the intensive care nursery would have to undergo for days, weeks—perhaps months. Parents had no one except busy doctors and overworked nurses to explain to them what was happening, and there was absolutely no one to offer help and support.

This book offers help, support, and information for "preemie" parents. It gives an "insider's view," an intimate picture for social workers, nurses, and doctors who become involved with not just a baby, but with a whole family. For those who are in (or plan to enter) social work, nursing, or medicine, we hope the book provides information, and more important, insight into the human beings you will be working with. For parents-to-be who hope for a normal, full-term pregnancy, Falecia and we hope along with you. But we also believe that we will have done something for you just in case your hopes, and our hopes, are not met.

Dr. Bernard Griesemer

Fred and Faye Pfister

Falecia Pfister

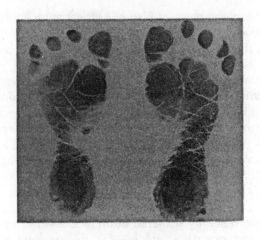

ACKNOWLEDGMENTS

If we were to acknowledge all those who helped with and contributed in some manner to this book, its length would be doubled. Let it suffice that the thousands of parents of preemies are to be thanked—for their ideas, suggestions, questions, and contributions.

The Nursing Staff at the Lester E. Cox Intensive Care Nursery certainly must be thanked for all their help, suggestions, and inspiration—as well as their care of Falecia, who inspired the book. Dana Wells and the Public Relations Department of Cox have also been very helpful. Lynne A. Lumsden of Prentice-Hall's General Publishing Division is to be thanked for her revision suggestions, as is her editorial assistant Bill Cosco, who provided answers to our many questions.

And finally, a debt of gratitude goes to Cindy Jones and Charlotte Rains for typing and retyping the manuscript (and for babysitting), and to Arleen Rand for her proofreading.

Our thanks to you all.

Fred Pfister

Bernard Griesemer

THE LITTLEST BABY

chapter one

WHY ME? INITIAL QUESTIONS AND FEARS

A PARENT SPEAKS

This is my story. It could just as easily be yours. It could be the story of any of the thousands who each year find themselves the parents of a premature child. Each story would be different, but each story would have the same feelings and fears, the same soul-searching, the same questioning, and the same questions.

I'm writing about myself because I want to try to understand myself—that's why most people write about themselves. People read about the lives of others because they are able to put the astounding fact of their own lives in better perspective. All lives are fantastic to those who have not lived them, and those reading this book may have an equally fantastic story that is just as good—perhaps even better because it would be their very own.

Some of the stories about nature's littlest miracles turn out to be tragedies. Others end happily, but all are part of the great drama of life, and not a single scene or line can be altered after it is played.

And how does my story end? Who knows? It is still being written. Each day adds another page to the drama in which I and the people I know are players. Before I actually begin, I should correct myself. It's not *my* story. It's *our* story—my wife's and mine. It just happens to be told from my point of view.

Where do I begin? Perhaps I should follow Alice's advice in *Through the Looking Glass:* "Start at the beginning, proceed until you come to the middle, and continue until you get to the end." That advice, however, is difficult to follow. When a parent becomes involved in the events connected with having a premature child, there seems to be no logical order to life. Things just happen. You seem to have no control. A thousand questions come to mind, and those who can answer—doctors and nurses—are often so busy that they can't take time to answer. Just as bad, perhaps even worse, you don't know *what* to ask. You just have fears, doubts, and concerns that can't find expression, and your mind jumps on the proverbial horse and goes galloping off in a dozen directions at once. Because every case is different, and because parents carry their own individual backgrounds as intellectual baggage, the questions they would ask and the order they would ask them will be different.

In telling our story, I will interrupt from time to time to pose those questions I did ask, that I wanted to ask, or that other parents have told me they wanted to ask. Reflecting on the events, Dr. Griesemer can provide the answers in an informative, unhurried "bedside manner" that he may not be able to do in real life because of the hectic pace of a profession in which life and death situations and crises are commonplace.

So to begin at the beginning . . .

I suppose the real beginning would have been a walk in November—November 22 to be exact, or at least so we think. Faye and I were visiting my parents for the Thanksgiving holiday and my mother's birthday. We decided to walk over their farm and several neighboring farms after a huge dinner. (My mother could never get out of the habit of cooking for six boys.) The air was crisp but not biting, and the sky seemed almost a summertime blue. It was not at all like Thanksgiving weather. Only the trees, stark and bare, would have us believe it was fall.

After a walk of several miles through fields of fescue and broomsage, and across creeks, we stopped to rest in a pine grove. Seated on the carpet of pine needles, our talk led to a kiss, kisses led to caresses, and then all I remember is Faye's black hair and white skin against the textured pine needles.

We took no precautions. But for the last ten years we hadn't. When we were first married and I was going to graduate school and Faye was teaching, she had taken the pill. When we had decided to start a family and quit the preventatives, nothing happened. And nothing continued to happen. We kept thinking, "Well, if it does, it does. But we are happy enough without any children."

And so we continued our work and our education. Faye earned a Master of Fine Arts degree and taught art in the public school, and I got my advanced degrees in English. I accepted a position at a small, private liberal arts school in the Ozarks, a picture postcard college with limestone buildings and a Gothic cathedral covered with ivy set atop a big bluff overlooking the meandering White River and a broad valley. The area is the Midwest Mecca for tourists, who come to vacation in the heart of Ozark Mountain Country.

Ten months before that Thanksgiving walk, while I was conducting a group of students on a tour of London, Faye's routine Pap test had come back positive. After I got back, "belly button surgery" was scheduled, and the cell growth in her uterus was found to be premalignant. The doctor told us not to worry, but he suggested that the abnormal tissue be checked again. If it became worse, Faye was to have her uterus removed.

Faye was scheduled to have a D & C in December during her school's Christmas break, the day after Christmas. But the D & C to check on the growth of the premalignancy was an operation that was not to be. And so this is the way the story begins, I think. At least that is the way I would like to think it began—in the pine grove, green needles against blue sky, the soft shag carpet of brown, on my mother's birthday that crisp November afternoon.

In early December, Faye thought she was pregnant, and I, of course, just laughed. Such a possibility was too fantastic, too remote, and although she bulged out of every bra she had, neither of us *really* believed she could be pregnant. Christmas was coming fast, it was the end of the semester, and we had finals and final grades to worry about. I was busy with my classes, and Faye was busy with hers.

When Christmas vacation began, we had time to really think about ourselves instead of our students and school. A good friend, Patty, had been privy to our speculations, and she was even more curious than we were. She insisted that we find out for sure. "As your Christmas present, I'm going to get you a home pregnancy test kit," she said to Faye one evening after dinner. We had come out of our small town's main street cafe, and the Christmas shoppers swirled past like so many brightly colored snowflakes. Patty marched across the street to the drugstore and returned a few minutes later with the kit.

"You should have seen the look he gave me when I bought this," she giggled. "My diamondless hand really must have made him wonder. I'll be the subject of the town's gossip for at least the next week!" She almost seemed to gloat at the prospect.

The test kit was supposed to make a tiny doughnut in two hours to show a pregnancy. In less than two hours, a definite doughnut shape was visible. There was no doubt. Our remotest suspicions were confirmed. Our jokes and jests could be put aside. We immediately began counting backwards to find out when the whole thing had occurred (that's when the November date was decided on), and then forward to see when we could expect the big event. It would be the middle of August. A Leo—courageous and lionhearted. That was good. I had two brothers born in that month, and Faye and I had been married in August.

We decided not to tell anyone the news until Faye's doctor had given her the rabbit test. Faye's doctor already had the hospital scheduled for the D & C surgery when Faye mentioned to him that she might be pregnant. An examination convinced him, but he ordered a lab test just to confirm his diagnosis. It also was positive. We could now tell the world.

At first, nobody would believe us. All of our friends our own age had children who were in school, and some even had children who would be graduating from high school in the spring. They were all amazed and pleased. I'm a bit puzzled about this, but most people think your life isn't really complete until you have had children. They may be right. We had always been perfectly satisfied before, but our news seemed like icing on the cake.

The New Year's Eve parties were exciting, and the announcement of a new year's baby gladdened everybody. New Year's Day, we called friends far and wide—an actor friend in Hawaii, and an artist friend in Taiwan who had some news of his own. He too expected a child in August. He was so excited, and his English was so rusty, we could barely communicate!

From the moment we heard our news, we knew what names we wanted. We decided that if it were a boy, it would be named Fredrick Rolla, after my father and me, and a girl would be named Falecia Jean, a combination of sounds in Faye's name, her mother's middle name, Lee, and my mother's name, Jean. We had decided to change the spelling from the more common Felecia, which comes from the Latin *felicitas* (happy).

We decided that Faye would spend a year at home with the baby, and although it would be rough financially, we began preparing for the year that we would be living only on my salary. Faye wrote a letter to her school board, asking for a year's leave of absence. The reason for her request rather surprised them, but they were more than glad to grant it.

The new year was going well. Faye had been granted her leave of absence, I had gotten several articles accepted by professional journals, and I was to present two papers at national professional meetings. It was going to be a good year. But the best laid plans of mice and men go astray. In April, everything suddenly changed.

On the twelfth, a Saturday, I returned from a professional meeting just in time for us to attend a combination party and film. A group at school had formed a film club of sorts, with a different member hosting a film at his or her house each month. This month was a French film *Jules and Jim*, and my school's French professor was providing the drinks and her home as the theatre.

During the film, Faye felt uncomfortable, and left the den to lie down on a bed. We left shortly afterward, missing most of the food, drink, and chitchat. Faye said she had gone to the bathroom and noticed a good deal of blood and had felt "a balloon" above her vaginal vault. The next day Faye wasn't better, and the spotting of blood that had started the night before continued. So at her doctor's suggestion, she stayed in bed all day Sunday. Her next regular appointment was scheduled for Tuesday, but we decided that she should see her doctor in Springfield, a forty-eight mile drive, Monday. Faye arranged for a substitute to take her art classes, and Patty, who was now as interested in the pregnancy as if it were her very own, agreed to go with her.

My Monday classes were draggy—the students seemed to have partied all weekend—and I felt I didn't do much myself to make class lively. My mind wasn't on my lectures or the material at hand. I could hardly wait for the day to end, so I could get home to find out the news of Faye. I didn't have to wait that long.

My secretary interrupted me in my two o'clock class and told me that Faye had called and had broken down on the phone, saying that she had to be admitted to the hospital. The secretary spoke in a low, hushed voice at the door, but my students, who had paid little enough attention earlier, seemed to have grown ears to overhear the conversation.

I'm the kind of teacher who believes, and likes to have others believe, that nothing is more important than my class. After all, I tell my students the only legitimate reasons for ever missing class are having a baby or death. But it took me only seconds to announce, "Continued next time," and make an assignment.

The forty-eight-mile drive to the hospital was slowed by the incoming tourist traffic. It probably seemed slower than it really was, but it gave me time to think. The events in which I was participating—which I felt were *happening* to me because I had no control—were totally unexpected. I had expected Faye to have a normal pregnancy, to have a normal delivery of a normal, healthy child. I had, like a true Capricorn, scheduled everything. A miscarriage was not on the schedule, and so it took some rearrangement in my thinking. The baby meant lots, but it didn't mean as much as Faye.

I expected the worst, but when I got to the hospital, I found Faye smiling in her dress, on the hospital bed, answering the usual inane admittance questions. "Do you have any jewelry? Do you have any insurance?" Patty looked just as comfortable. It was nothing at all like I had built it up to be in my mind. Faye was still obviously pregnant—no blood, no tears, no miscarriage.

Between the nurse's questions, Faye told me what her doctor had said. She had gone into labor at the film because of an incompetent cervix. It wouldn't support the weight of the baby, and she had actually dilated to four centimeters, almost half of what is necessary for a normal delivery. The "balloon" she had felt was the amniotic sack. The doctor was amazed that Faye hadn't miscarried.

Before I could assimilate all the information, her room phone rang. I answered, thinking it would be for the nurse. It was for me. I was amazed. It was Faye's sister, and I wondered how she had known we were at the hospital. I found out—and I found out the bad news. She had called my office on campus, and my secretary told her that I had gone to the hospital to see Faye. The reason she was calling was to tell us that Faye's 17-year-old nephew had killed himself after breaking up with his girlfriend. Bad news travels in a pack, I thought as I listened, wondering how to tell Faye.

Faye took it well. What could she do? She seemed emotionally numb as she told me that the doctor was prescribing a drug, Brethine, to stop the premature labor contractions. Her cervix would have to be sutured—sewn up—to support the weight of the baby. Faye would have to remain in bed for the rest of the pregnancy.

What a way to spend summer vacation, I thought. But what else could we do? Faye immediately began lesson plans for the substitute teacher who would finish her art classes. I called Faye's superintendent that night, and he made arrangements for her replacement, pointing out that she probably had enough accumulated sick days to avoid losing the rest of her salary. His almost parental concern was nice; a small school in a small town encourages that sort of down-home, human relationship.

Faye's cervix surgery was scheduled for nine o'clock Thursday. I had never heard of such a procedure before, but the wife of a colleague in the political science department knew all about it and even produced an article she had recently read about it. I couldn't be in Springfield that day at all, and I felt rather guilty about it. That was the day I had scheduled a Creative Writing Workshop/Contest for area high school students, and a swarm of 300 aspiring writers were on campus. At nine o'clock I was listening to the college's Act I Players read some of the student selections. They were often gushy love lyrics and I intellectually pooh-poohed their sentimentality, but my heart closed the gap between Faye and me. And then I thought of her nephew, whose funeral had been the previous day. Some of the students here today had attended. Perhaps these writers knew more of life than I gave them credit for.

I was gratified to see students from Faye's school, and many of the students she had in art class, sweep the contest portion of the event. And at the awards assembly that afternoon, one of her students slipped me a card to give to Faye. She had it before an hour had passed after the event was over. Faye had gone through the surgery in fine form. She was smiling when I handed her the card and told her about her school's fine performance.

Hospital rest helped, but Faye continued to have vaginal bleeding after being up on her feet for only a few minutes. Her doctor told her the next Tuesday that she could go home, but that she would have to stay in bed.

By now, Faye's pregnancy and its complications had become a community affair. Friends brought her lunch while I was in class, and there was always enough for dinner after I got home. Our Sunday school class bought her a wicker bed tray, complete with glass holder and magazine rack. Another neighbor, the block's "professional mother" in whose yard the neighbor children always played, checked in periodically, and I had a phone installed next to the bed so friends could call.

Despite such help and conveniences, it was going to be a long summer. My semester was about to end, and I would have to be getting ready for term papers and finals. There would be no summer vacation, because I had contracted to teach during the summer session. In addition to my classes, I was busy with an area Arts and Cultural Committee that had arranged a community concert in the college's fieldhouse that Sunday—a dulcimer orchestra, a symphony orchestra, and a chorus of 350 voices drawn from local church choirs. I felt rather guilty because I hadn't done as much work as I thought I should have for the event, but I was looking forward to it. Carol, an Arkansas friend we had gone to college with, had come up to spend the weekend with us and attend the concert, but she stayed home to keep Faye company.

The night before the concert, Faye complained about her stomach, and she had a thick, yellowish discharge. Sunday, she was worse, and a nurse in our Sunday school class suggested that I take her to the hospital. She suspected that her "waters had broken." I asked John, a friend who taught in the Sociology Department, to borrow his station wagon. He had offered it before to use as an ambulance. He thought our ten-year-old Volkswagen rode rough, and Faye certainly didn't need to make the trip to the hospital again in our VW.

Carol was beside herself, and seemed dazed as we repacked Faye's suitcase. She had come, expecting a concert and conversation, adapted to a bedridden Faye, and found herself in the middle of our crisis. After John came with his station wagon, Carol brought Faye's suitcase and belongings while I picked Faye up from the bed. Her normal weight was 112; her top weight during the pregnancy had been 118, and judging from the heft of her, she certainly didn't weigh any more than that. In fact, she seemed to weigh less than the 100-pound sacks of dairy feed I had so often handled on my parents' farm.

I carefully placed Faye in the back of the station wagon. Carol gave her a blanket and pillow, and then burst into tears. She wasn't going to go with us, she hated hospitals because they made her cry. I told Carol I would call her after we arrived. Faye, who had remained calm all morning, started crying when Carol started, and John, who had brought a few remaining things, just looked amazed. I wondered what a sociologist thought of the whole situation.

I turned on the car's emergency flasher, hoping it would cause some of the gawking tourists to pull over as we raced north on Highway 65. I was thankful for the new road. The forty-eight-mile trip was now a breeze—no twenty mph curves like old 65, which had followed the ridges and had snaked around our mountains in the Ozarks. We made the trip in record time. I hadn't realized how much speed our VW lost going up hills until I drove something that maintained constant speed, no matter what the load or grade. We pulled into the ambulance area of the hospital, where a nurse was waiting. Carol had called, telling them to expect us.

It was now almost eleven o'clock, and Faye was made comfortable, if such a word can be used, in one of the labor rooms of the maternity ward. There wasn't anything I could do except wait. A preliminary examination confirmed our worst fears. The amniotic sack had broken. The yellowish discharge had been the amniotic fluid, which had become infected, probably as the result of last week's surgery. Faye would have to have the baby—she would have to miscarry. She had gained so little weight. In fact, Faye hadn't even worn maternity clothes.

I sat down with Faye in the labor room and prepared myself for the ordeal. The hours dragged on. The baby's heartbeat was checked regularly, and it continued to be stable and strong. Faye complained that she was hot. In fact, she had a 103° fever, and she would not dilate. I thought it was cold, and I wrapped myself up in a blanket one of the nurses brought in. The nurse was sympathetic and helpful—and also pregnant. She was about as far along as Faye.

The only time I ever got warm was when I watched the nurse on the next shift put an IV into Faye. She had trouble finding a vein, and Faye's pain and writhing made me feel faint. I broke out in a sweat and had to sit down.

There was little conversation between us. Her discomfort made conversation virtually impossible, but there was that wordless communication of comfort and concern that can only exist between two who know each other well, who are able to read paragraphs into a look or a gesture.

Time passed slowly. There was a knock at the door, and when I answered, it was Faye's mother. A genuine hill woman, she had raised thirteen children, and her mother had been a granny woman—an Ozarks midwife. She and one of her daughters-in-law had gone to visit Faye, and they were a bit shocked to find us gone and only Carol there. After learning the situation, they came directly to the hospital.

Faye's contractions were widely spaced, and so the women chitchatted. I was amazed they could be so calm. I felt helpless, and I tried to make myself useful by bathing Faye's forehead with cold wash cloths.

The afternoon wore on. Janet and Suzanne, two professors' wives, came in to visit. They gave Faye ice, and massaged her back. At 9:10 P.M., Faye had dilated enough, and she was wheeled into the delivery room. I scrubbed, and gowned myself, and followed.

Faye's doctor was out of town, and so one of his colleagues took on the delivery. Dr. Bernard Griesemer, the pediatrician on call, was standing by. Springfield, a city of 150,000, had no neonatologist. I had never met Dr. Griesemer, and never heard of him. Faye and I were putting our trust in a total stranger. I, a person who liked to think I made things happen, who liked to believe I had control over my life, found myself without control. Things were happening so fast I had no time to think about them, and no time to ask questions of those who may have had some control over the events.

The delivery was over in minutes. At 9:30 P.M., the doctor held up the tiny, kicking being—in one hand. "A girl," he announced. Under the glaring, hot lights all I saw was a small redness, and some frail movement. She was weighed, placed for only a moment on the scale, and rushed from the room to Dr. Griesemer. "Seven hundred grams," the nurse announced. My mind, not used to thinking in grams, raced to more familiar figures. She weighed less than two pounds—in fact, a pound and a half. There was no hope for her to survive. It was all I could do to hide my disappointment.

A DOCTOR SPEAKS

When Fred Pfister and I talked about preparing this handbook, compiling the questions he asked, the questions he wanted to ask, and the questions other parents have asked, we faced time and space restrictions that precluded an all-inclusive review of the field of neonatology. In addition, we talked about the concern parents and the public have about premature children. Often the public's interest borders on the same kind of curiosity that attracts people to a circus sideshow or to the *Guinness Book of World Records*. A parent, on the other hand, shows more human concern. Parents seek information that will help them and their premature child.

The questions that Falecia caused in the minds of the Pfisters are, I believe, typical. The answers, I hope, will provide information and help not just for the parents of premature children and their relatives, but also soon-to-be parents, doctors, nurses, and social workers.

1. What is prematurity?

Prematurity is abnormal, and before we can talk about what isn't normal, we need to know what is normal. The normal human pregnancy actually lasts thirty-eight to forty-two weeks. Technically, any child born before the thirty-eighth week of confinement in the womb is considered a pre-term baby. The technical term for a mother's due date is the "EDC" (Estimated Date of Confinement). With new ultrasound scanning, the accuracy of the EDC is becoming more and more precise.

At one time, all low-weight babies were thought to be preterm. Now doctors know it is not weight but time in the womb that defines a pre-term. Some pre-term babies weigh as much as 5 lbs. 8 oz. Full-term babies may weigh less than 5 lbs., and yet be physically mature enough to breathe and suck normally shortly after birth, functions with which pre-term babies often have difficulty. Because these babies are born too soon, many of their biological systems, such as those involving the lungs and liver, are not developed enough to work properly on their own. This can result in jaundice or breathing difficulties after birth. Usually children less than thirty-six weeks gestation (length of pregnancy) are the premature infants who have the most problems. The youngest infant likely to survive, when born premature, is twenty-four to twenty-six weeks.

Although biological immaturity is the main concern in caring for pre-term babies, weight also indicates how well a baby will do after birth. The smaller the baby, the greater the risks involved and the more intensive the care required.

What is confusing to many parents is their first encounter with a premature infant. What should they expect, how will they react to their baby, and how will their baby react to them?

2. Is prematurity common?

More common than most people believe. Dr. Irwin Merkatiz, an obstetrical perinatologist, says that "preterm delivery is the single biggest problem in obstetrics today." Nearly 10 percent of white babies and 20 percent of black babies are born prematurely.

Estimates differ, but it is generally believed that about one in every seven of the 3.3 million infants born each year in the United States is a high risk baby that either has a low birth weight or is premature. Just as estimates differ nationally, prematurity figures vary from region to region and even from city to city. A recent study by the Robert Wood Johnson Foundation found that an estimated 27.5 percent of babies born in Arizona would be classified as high risk babies, but only 10 percent of the babies born in Cleveland, Ohio would fall in that category.

So it can be said that a larger number of babies than most people would believe are born prematurely each year in the United States. Falecia's case may be unusual because of her extreme prematurity, but prematurity itself is common. Also, prematurity is responsible for three out of four newborn deaths.

3. What causes some babies to be born prematurely?

In many cases, we don't know why. There are, however, some very clear causes for a child to be born premature. First, there may be problems with the placenta (afterbirth), the organ that nourishes the baby during pregnancy. Trauma that causes separation of the placenta from the wall of the uterus (abruptio placentae) will routinely start a woman's labor and subsequent birth. The mother's placenta may be located in the lower rather than the upper portion of the uterus (placenta previa). An infection in the placenta also can cause a baby to be born prematurely. Poor nutrition can cause a very small placenta, and a small placenta is more prone to malfunction. Even if the placenta is normal, smoking, alcohol, and "recreational drugs" can interfere with the baby's development. Women who use such substances have a greater incidence of prematurity.

Secondly, a mother's physical problems can often cause premature labor. For example, mothers who are diabetic or have high blood pressure before or during pregnancy are more prone to give birth prematurely.

According to Dr. Carl A. Keller, an epidemiologist with the National Institute of Health, the most accurate predictor of pre-term birth is the mother's past obstetrical history. Women with histories of difficult pregnancies, spontaneous abortions, or stillbirths are more apt to give birth prematurely than women who have had full-term babies. So are women who have multiple pregnancy (twins, triplets, and so on). But the reason some women cannot carry to full term is not always clear: The cause may be biological, chemical, genetic, or a combination of factors.

The incidence of pre-term and low-weight babies is higher among teen-agers than other age groups. This greater risk may be caused by simple physical immaturity. Improper diet and inadequate medical care are major contributors to pre-term and low-weight birth, no matter what age the mother.

In about 50 percent of the cases, a doctor won't be able to give a specific cause. When a doctor can't give a specific reason, the mother often blames herself—for having sex during pregnancy, working, taking a trip, or exercising vigorously during the pregnancy. These are not causes of premature delivery, and if as a parent you find your mind dwelling on fixing the blame, further discussion with your doctor may be helpful.

In Falecia's case, her premature delivery was not caused by any one single problem. A major factor was the premature dilation of her mother's cervix—an incompetent cervix. This term, although technically correct and neutral sounding for a doctor, tends to explode in a mother's mind. Further explanation of the anatomy and physiology involved, and the fact that mothers can neither cause nor prevent an incompetent cervix, can alleviate some of the anguish many mothers experience.

Most anxieties are caused by fear of the unknown. A little bit of explanation will do much to decrease a mother's worries and guilt feelings. But in order for you to get that explanation, you must ask. Doctors don't read minds, and most doctors think that patients who ask questions are the best patients to have. When in doubt, always ask.

4. Is there anything that can be done to prevent a woman from having premature delivery?

Doctors have tried to prevent or halt early labor by various means— bed rest, sewing up the cervix (both were tried on Falecia's mother), prescribing sedatives, giving various hormone inhibitors, and even prescribing alcohol.

Recently a drug has been successful in delaying labor long enough to allow a baby to mature sufficiently to survive outside the womb. This new drug, Ritodrine, has successfully prolonged pregnancy to the thirty-sixth week in many cases. However, its uses are somewhat restricted. It cannot be used on women with hypertension or heart conditions, nor can it be used for pregnancies in which the placenta has separated from the uterus or those in which the amniotic sac has broken and become infected. Also, if delivery is expected shortly, Ritodrine cannot be used. In addition to Ritodrine, there are other drugs that are currently used experimentally. At the time of Falecia's birth, one of these—Brethine—was used.

A major issue that often faces doctors is whether to prescribe drugs for women during pregnancy. Women with chronic medical problems may need to take drugs on a regular basis, while some women require medication to treat conditions caused by the pregnancy. Others may need drugs to initiate or maintain the pregnancy. Contrary to past belief that the placenta protects the unborn infant from most drugs taken by the mother, there is now evidence that many drugs are passed from mother to child through the placenta. Because of the difficulties involved in testing the effect of prescription drugs on the human fetus, questions about their potential harm or safety remain unanswered. More research is needed to determine how safe various drugs are, and until such findings are available, pregnant women should take drugs only when necessary and only under a doctor's care.

5. What is the youngest premature baby born to have survived?

That is a difficult question. The problem is with the word *youngest.* When a baby is born, usually the doctor and the mother are not sure how old the baby is. Even if the mother knows precisely the day of conception, the development of a baby in the womb can vary considerably from mother to mother and from fetus to fetus.

As we have already mentioned, before a baby is born doctors can estimate its age by studying an ultrasound picture of the baby's head and comparing the measurement of it with a growth chart. By ultrasound, it is even possible for the mother to see a TV picture of the fetus. We can also snap a picture of the unborn child.

After the baby is born, doctors can estimate its age using a measurement of its head. This is the most accurate determination of a premature infant's true gestational age. It is called the Dubowitz test. It assesses multiple areas of fetal/infant development and is accurate to within one week of the baby's true age.

6. What is the smallest baby to have survived?

Now we are talking about something that can be accurately measured, but the figures can be deceptive. A 3 lb. baby may be older and more mature, and thus have a greater chance of surviving, than a 4 lb. baby in the next incubator. There are many factors that contribute to smallness, or low birth weight—the age of the baby, nutrition, placenta development, and other factors. There have been full-term babies weighing less than three pounds.

The *Guinness Book of World Records* lists the smallest baby to have survived as a 10 oz. 12¼-inch baby born unattended June 5,

1938. She was fed every hour through a fountain pen filler. It also reports a 12 oz. baby born Feb. 20, 1936 in Illinois as the smallest documented infant to survive in the United States.

Recently there was a report of a 460-gram baby, or 1.01 pounds, who was born fourteen weeks prematurely on November 29, 1979. That would make Russell Ordell Williams the smallest baby to have survived in the U.S., who developed normally. But by the time you read this information, with all the advances being made in medical technology and neonatology, this information will probably be out of date. For example, as small as Falecia was, and as young as she is, she has already been replaced as the smallest surviving infant born at that particular hospital. That baby is already at home, doing well, and waiting to be replaced by another record breaker.

In recent years, revolutionary advances have been made in the care of pre-term babies. With the help of medical technology, babies born at or before twenty-seven weeks and weighing less than 2 lbs. often survive. More importantly, those who survive have greater probability of growing up to be normal and healthy children.

7. Can the use of drugs, or even coffee and alcohol, cause prematurity?

It is a rule of thumb that a poorly developed placenta may cause prematurity. Anything that a mother does that interferes with the growth and development of the placenta, and its ability to provide food and oxygen to her baby, increases the chances of prematurity. The old saying, "You are what you eat" can be revised for mothers to be, "Your baby eats and drinks and smokes what you eat and drink and smoke."

Mothers who smoke, mothers who ingest large amounts of alcohol, and mothers who use "recreational drugs" are more prone to have a premature baby than mothers who avoid such substances. These substances can cause problems with the placenta and its development, and certainly they are damaging to the developing baby.

According to the 1979 Report of the Surgeon General, the risk of miscarriage and infant death increases directly with increased levels of smoking during pregnancy. Because smoking is associated with low birthweight, it is best for pregnant women to stop or reduce smoking. It is known that more poor women who smoke have low-weight babies than do women in higher economic brackets who smoke. Perhaps certain conditions associated with low birthweight and poverty—inadequate nutrition and medical care—are compounded by the effects of tobacco. Cigarette smoking decreases the oxygen supply to the placenta and, hence, to the baby. The nicotine is transfused to the baby's system, and one cigarette can actually raise the heart beat of the fetus by five beats per minute.

Alcohol in large quantities is generally not healthy, and it stands to reason that it would not be good for a developing baby. The THC in marijuana, like any substance that will be carried in the blood, will be transferred through the membrane between mother and baby. Recent research findings show that babies of drug addicted and alcoholic mothers are more likely to be born pre-term, suffer birth defects, and often even undergo drug withdrawal immediately after birth.

Although the effects of many prescription drugs are not known, some should definitely not be taken during pregnancy. The benefits and the potential risks of specific drugs should be discussed with your physician. It is important to inform your physician if you are pregnant, or better yet, discuss what medications you are taking *before* you become pregnant.

Sometimes it is even helpful if your obstetrician knows which drugs your parents took. For example, between 1940 and 1970 a synthetic hormone called diethylstilbestrol (DES) was prescribed for women who were thought to be likely to miscarry. There is recent research that shows that the daughters of women who took this drug have an unusually high rate of late miscarriage, ectopic pregnancy (a condition in which the fetus is implanted in the fallopian tube instead of the uterus), and premature birth.

Recently, doctors have also become very concerned with industrial pollutants and the effect they may have on pregnancy and breast-feeding. Substances such as DDT, PCB's, and so on are now undergoing intensive monitoring by private and governmental agencies. A conscientious mother will watch carefully what she ingests, not only to prevent the possibility of prematurity, but also to increase her chances of having a normal, healthy, well-developed baby.

8. Is prematurity inherited?

No, prematurity is not inherited, but some of the conditions that can cause it are inherited. For example, there is a tendency for diabetes to recur in a family. If such a condition occurs in your family, then your chances of having a premature child are greatly increased. However, good prenatal care is the most significant factor in reducing the risks for parents who may have inherited conditions which make them high risk cases for prematurity.

9. If my first child was born prematurely, does this mean that if I have other children, they will also be premature?

Statistically, mothers who have previous miscarriages and premature infants are more prone to have further premature deliveries. Your risk is determined more on the basis of the causes of the first child being premature. For instance, if a mother has problems with her womb that cause her first baby to be premature, and that problem cannot be corrected, her subsequent children may also be premature.

Proper medical care is the best way to ensure a mother's health and her baby's welfare, although there are cases where doctors cannot solve the mysteries of difficult pregnancy or pre-term birth. From the time a woman suspects she is pregnant until she gives birth, she should have regular obstetrical examinations.

10. If young mothers often have premature babies, what about older mothers?

This question is becoming more common in the last three or four years. With many American women now planning their children around their careers, or waiting to have children until they are near thirty or even older, the question arises much more often. And it will become more frequent as the large age group of women between twenty-seven and thirty-seven plan families.

An "older woman" who is planning to have a child has no greater risk of bearing a premature child than a woman in the 20–25 age group, unless she has a documented history of miscarriages. But all available studies show that prematurity is the least of a mature woman's problems. There are, however, other problems she must face—the greatest is simply getting pregnant. What may have worried her when she conscientiously practiced birth control may now be difficult to accomplish. The fertility rate for women over twenty-seven drops dramatically. And if an older woman does get pregnant, the risks of having a baby with a genetic defect, such as Down's syndrome, increases.

Falecia's mother, for example, postponed a family until she was in her mid-30's, and had some difficulty getting pregnant. Never having had a history of miscarriages, she never dreamed of having a preemie, but did worry about having a Down's syndrome baby. As it turned out, she was one of those cases in which no single reason can be given for the premature birth, although an incompetent cervix was implicated, but her age had little to do with the prematurity.

So the woman who has postponed getting pregnant for a number of years faces certain problems, but prematurity is not necessarily one of them.

11. My doctor says that the twins I am carrying are likely to be born prematurely. How does my doctor know that?

Most multiple birth babies are born prematurely. It may be nature's way of protecting the mother, to keep the babies from overtaxing her body. In some cases, inducing premature delivery is necessary because the doctor believes the babies' chances of survival outside the womb are better than their chances if they are carried to full term. Although nothing is ever certain in medicine, your physician will be relatively confident that the babies will be old enough and mature enough to face up to the rigors of life outside the womb. Newer techniques in ultrasound and in analysis of the amniotic fluid (obtained by amniocentesis) have proved to be invaluable aids in determining the safest time for delivery.

If you are carrying twins or triplets, your physician may recommend that the babies be born by Caesarean section. This procedure minimizes birth trauma for the babies and maximizes their chances for survival.

12. My doctor says that the baby I am carrying has a problem that can be solved by in-womb surgery. Is that possible?

It is possible, and as technology improves, it will probably be more common. Until recently, a woman who knew she was carrying a child with an abnormality had two choices: therapeutic abortion or having a child who would be doomed to an early death, or severe physical or mental problems. Now there may be, at least for certain disorders, a third choice—the correction of the defect while the baby is still developing in its mother's womb.

In-womb surgery is done with sonar techniques developed to find submerged submarines. Ultrasound, as it is called, bounces sound waves off an object, in this case the unborn baby, giving a picture of the baby. The ultrasound machinery, which is much like a depth gauge on a boat, creates images of the fetus on a television screen. Still and motion pictures can be made of the fetus, and in the "motion machine," fetal motions are seen as they occur. Ultrasound waves, unlike X-rays, are currently regarded as being very safe. Using ultrasound, doctors can establish the gestational age of the fetus, they can determine if there is more than one fetus, and, more important, they can detect many abnormalities in both the fetus and placenta.

The developments in the field of *in-utero* surgery are probably one of the most exciting and promising areas of medicine. Currently, only collapsed lungs, Rh disease, urinary tract obstruction, enzyme-deficiency diseases, thyroid deficiency, and the buildup of excess fluid in the brain, lungs, and abdomen can be treated.

But recently, there have been exciting developments. At the Colorado Health Sciences Center, a delicate brain operation was developed to drain fluid from the brain of a fetus that suffered from hydrocephalus, a condition that causes excess fluid to accumulate in the brain cavity, preventing the brain from developing normally because of the buildup of pressure. The surgery consisted of inserting a miniature tube to provide a drain of the fluid from the brain into the amniotic fluid. This allowed the brain to develop normally, and after birth, another draining tube was inserted to divert the fluid from the brain into the abdomen.

Not only can doctors drain fluids, they can also infuse fluids into the fetus. The most notable example of this is when there is an Rh-blood incompatibility between the mother and the baby. In the past, doctors had to wait until the baby was born to make the needed blood change. However, many babies died during birth or shortly afterward, and it was decided that it might be better to give the transfusion before the birth, by inserting a needle carrying red blood cells through the mother's abdomen.

Such dramatic surgery will, as techniques and technology improve, become more common. But Dr. Gary Hodgen, chief of the Pregnancy Research Branch of the National Institutes of Health warns, "It's important not to give expectant parents false hopes. Even if we can diagnose and repair an abnormality, the affected child may have multiple malformations that cannot be corrected." Of course any such surgery is risky and could result in premature delivery. It is used only if it is absolutely needed.

13. Are more boy babies or girl babies born prematurely? Which has the better chance of surviving?

More males are born prematurely than females, perhaps only because there are more males born than females in normal, full-term pregnancies. So, the chances of having a premature boy or a girl are no greater than the chances in a normal pregnancy. The fact that more males are born than females may be Nature's way of compensating for the fact that more males succumb to disease, war, and accidents.

In the case of premature babies, the chances of survival are better for girls. No one really knows why. They may mature earlier in the womb, just as they mature a bit earlier in adolescence. Many of my female colleagues feel they really are the stronger sex and have greater endurance. In any event, the survival rate for preemie girls is about 51 percent compared to 49 percent for preemie boys.

Nurses often comfort parents who have a girl preemie by telling them this fact. I suppose they don't say anything about the statistics when the patient is a boy. It is interesting to note that Falecia was the smallest baby to have survived at the hospital where she was born. Within a year, her record was broken by another preemie, also a girl.

14. Does a seven-month baby have a greater chance of surviving than an eight-month baby?

No, the belief that a seven-month baby is more likely to survive is an old wives' tale that just won't die. The less premature a baby is, the better chance it has to survive. Obviously, an eight-month baby is more mature than a seven-month baby.

Many parents are confused when they learn that some small babies may survive and larger babies may not. But many factors can affect the survival of infants. Although some children are in the 4-5 lb. category, they may be premature and have a higher risk of complications or death than older 3-4 lb. babies who are small because of intrauterine growth retardation. And being older, these babies' organs are more mature and able to withstand the stress placed on them.

The survival of any premature infant is often determined by the fact that if any one system goes wrong—a collapsed lung, for example—the stress it engenders causes problems in other systems. The collapsed lung may cause heart failure because the heart does not have enough reserve strength to endure the added strain.

Recently we have become increasingly aware of the fact that the premature infant's brain, and the blood vessels in and around the brain, are perhaps the most fragile of all the body systems. The most dreaded of all complications in the intensive care nursery is an *intracranial hemorrhage*, the premature infant's equivalent of a stroke. Oftentimes fatal, many times resulting in severe brain damage, difficult or impossible to prevent or treat, and shockingly rapid in onset and progression, its presence is far too common in babies weighing less than 1000 grams (2.2 lbs). The scene it creates is likewise far too common—a deteriorating infant, stunned parents, frustrated nurses, and doctors spending long, futile hours of work. Intracranial hemorrhage is a formidable foe and currently the subject of research in many centers.

15. How does the pediatrician or neonatologist and the ICN staff decide which premature babies they should try to save and which they should not?

That is a blunt question, and it demands an answer. It is very difficult, and there are so many factors to consider—the age, weight, and maturity of the premature baby, its "spirit and spunk," and how many problems and deformities it is born with. Every case must be decided on its own merits, and every one is a difficult decision.

The success rate for premature babies fewer than twenty-six weeks old and weighing fewer than 750 grams (about 2 lbs. 6 ozs.) is not good at all. And when these babies do survive, it is often with extensive damage. But the occasional survival of a very small premature baby catches the attention of people. The baby frequently receives wide coverage in the daily press and in popular magazines. The public is led to believe that it is possible for *every* premature baby to survive, no matter how small and immature.

You can imagine how this coverage puts pressure on doctors to save every baby, no matter how small. Add to that the pressures from Right to Life groups and the fears of malpractice suits, and neonatal units will have infants referred to them that weigh less than a pound and who have so little lung development that prolonged life outside the mother is practically impossible.

Such babies may survive for days, weeks, and months on machines, but they don't grow and develop, and they suffer extensive physical and mental damage. Because of their poor survival rate, generally a less aggressive, or "hands off," approach is followed. But hands off is not synonymous with "no care." The baby is kept warm, given oxygen, and heroic efforts are begun only at the request of the parents and only after the risks and benefits have been thoroughly explained to them.

A very small baby is, after all, a human being, and if it is too small and immature to survive, it has as much right to die with dignity as does any elderly patient.

16. I don't plan to have a premature delivery, but what can I do to plan ahead—just in case?

Of course no one deliberately plans to have a premature child. However, there are things a pregnant woman can be aware of that may save her child's life and herself grief.

Many mothers have had thoughts that their premature child would have survived had adequate medical facilities been available. Such thoughts are undoubtedly true, but not all hospitals have adequate facilities and not all cities and towns have populations large enough to be served by pediatricians and neonatologists. And just because you live in a sophisticated urban area is no guarantee that your premature child will receive the best care. Washington, D.C., for example, has had the worst, the second-worst, or third-worst infant mortality rate of any city in the country each year for the last decade. At first people were unconcerned, blaming the high rate on the large number of blacks, the high rate of teen-age pregnancy, and the often inadequate prenatal care of teen-ager mothers. But a study showed that these factors had little to do with the high infant mortality rate.

Another study of survival rates of premature children by the National Capital Medical Foundation showed that results vary widely from hospital to hospital. That study showed that more than 90 percent of the newborns who died in Washington that year weighed less than 2500 grams—high risk babies because of low birth weight or prematurity. The best hospital saved 54 percent of the babies weighing between 500 and 1000 grams. The next best hospital, one that middle class citizens would have thought would have had the best survivor rate because it was a private university teaching hospital, saved only 33 percent. A Washington, D.C. general hospital saved only 14 percent—a *mortality* rate of 86 percent!

In less-urbanized areas, the care for high risk children may be better, but it could just as easily be worse. Because the necessary skills of doctors and the necessary technology are so expensive, there are often only regional hospitals that can provide services for babies born very prematurely. If the baby is only slightly premature, most hospitals have adequate nursery care.

You might be interested in some of the Washington study's

findings. A shocking 14 percent of the babies who died were born, not in the hospital's delivery room, but in labor rooms, ward beds, and even hallways—as mothers waited for rooms. In an intensive study of 106 of those babies who weighed more than 500 grams, breathed for at least an hour, and had no lethal malformation, it was found that:

- Over 53 percent had not had a blood acidity test (p^H test)—a test needed to prescribe drugs.
- Almost 20 percent were blue (cyanotic) from a lack of oxygen in the blood and were not given oxygen in the ICN.
- Over 53 percent of the dead infants never had their blood pressure taken.
- Over 63 percent never had their blood sugar levels checked, a prerequisite for a doctor to decide what course of action should be taken.

Many of those 106 deaths were avoidable. Talk with your doctor about what he might do if you do have an excessively premature baby. Try to find out if he was trained in a time when physicians took the deaths of premature babies as natural, or a matter of course. Find the pediatricians or neonatologists practicing in your city. Ask questions.

To be on the safe side, you may check hospitals in your area. See what kind of facilities they have. If you have a history of pregnancy complications, know you are a high risk case, or know you expect twins or triplets it might be wise to plan delivery in a facility that has extensive neonatal expertise and facilities. Remember that most deliveries are not premature, but you can buy valuable time by checking ahead to see exactly what facilities are available.

If you live in a rural area, you may want to check what medical transport facilities are available. It is often possible to fly or rush a mother who has started labor prematurely to a hospital that has adequate facilities. More and more, as the cost of ICN care and technology increases, regional centers are being used, with rapid transportation from outlying areas by special ambulance or helicopter.

In the case of Falecia, her being born where she was greatly increased her chances of survival. Had she been born at home or in a hospital that lacked ICN facilities, she almost certainly would not have survived.

chapter two

YOU, THE NURSES, AND THE "MOTHER MACHINES"

A PARENT SPEAKS

I was now a father of a little girl, a very little girl, but I had no idea how many minutes she would live. I was a father, but there was no elation, no joy. I was a parent, but I had to put my trust for her survival in the hands of a virtual stranger.

I had talked with Dr. Griesemer earlier, and signed a form giving my "informed consent" for the necessary actions. He had said they would do what they could, but he emphasized that so much depended on the individual baby. I had had some hopes until I heard the nurse's pronouncement, "Seven hundred grams." The pound-and-a-half conversion figure struck me like a hammer blow. My glazed eyes stared at the antiseptic stainless steel landscape of the hospital.

I talked some minutes with Faye, and then I went to wait outside the intensive care nursery. I looked through the window. All the equipment inside was identified with a big *ICN* and a number. Dr. Griesemer came out and told me the news: Falecia was still alive and doing as well, even better than could be expected. He emphasized that the survival rate of "kilogram kids"—2.3 lbs. and under at birth—was not good. The odds for a baby her size, weight, and gestation length were one in a hundred. No poker player would bet on odds like that, but hope springs eternal in the human breast, and my stomach fluttered again, although I knew I shouldn't get my hopes up. I steeled myself, resolving not to get too attached so that if something went wrong, I wouldn't be hurt.

I went to see my first and only offspring, isolated in a room of her own because of the amniotic fluid infection, with a feeling of calculated detachment, a sense of emotional noninvolvement. The nurse directed me to the scrub room. The sign said, "Remove all jewelry. Scrub a full two minutes." I scrubbed an extra minute, resolving not to have a single germ on me that could make Falecia's fragile condition worse, and the brown medical soap and brush reddened my skin.

The spectacle of my daughter overwhelmed me—a wrinkled, wizened body, covered with fine hair so thick it seemed like fur. And her size! A baby shorter than my shoe! Pencil-sized arms and legs, waving madly. Patches and electrodes attached to her body, wires running to equipment I knew nothing about. Tubes running to her mouth, down her throat. Beeps and clicks and pulsating lights.

But they were all necessary. They were the machines that would mother her and care for her. Without an amniotic sac to protect her, without a placenta to feed her, to breathe for her, to oxygenate her blood, to eliminate her body waste, Falecia needed a "space suit" with all those wires and electrodes and tubes and needles. She was as close to death in this strange environment as I would be if I were suddenly transported to the surface of the moon. Being on the moon's surface without life support systems is no disease. Like an astronaut, she had been transported from an environment for which she had been perfectly adapted and thrust into an environment that could be deadly. Neither prayers nor technology could put her back into the uterus. For better or for worse, she was in this brave new world to stay.

The nurse knew that I too was a stranger in a strange land. She briefly explained what each alien machine was, the mothers that were to replace Faye. There was a heart monitor that let the nurses know her heart rate with an audible signal, a ventilator that breathed for her so many times a minute. She encouraged me to touch the hand-sized human, but I was reluctant. I was afraid I would "become attached" to her, and be doomed to the disappointment of her inexorable death. Besides, I was afraid that I would disconnect something, that she would break, that I might accidentally cause her harm, or even her death.

The nurse sensed my fears. She said that personal contact was important for both me and the baby. And she demonstrated that Falecia indeed wouldn't break. An audio alarm sounded on the other side of the ICN, calling her to some minor emergency with one of the nearly two dozen other infants, and she left us alone. Falecia was in a tiny room, isolated from all the other premature babies in the ICN, because of the amniotic fluid infection.

I gently stroked her leg with my little finger, a leg no bigger than my little finger. My wedding ring, I was sure, would slip on her leg past her knee. Her arms were the size of lead pencils, and both of them would have easily fit through my ring.

I bent closer. She had a fine head of hair and very long eyelashes. Her eyebrows were discernible, but just grew into a fine crop of "fur" that covered her forehead and merged with the thicker hair on her minute, but perfectly formed, teacup-sized head.

The continual flailings of her arms forced me to focus on her hands. I moved my little finger to her hand, and she grasped at it. Her hand, not much bigger than a nickel, could have never reached around my finger, but her grasp was strong and firm, like a handshake. The tips of her tiny fingers were bulbed, much like the enlarged fingers of a tree frog. They were white with the exertion of her grasp. If she were strong, I could be just as strong, but it would be her strength that would decide whether she lived or died.

I left, quietly closing the door. I went to see Faye. She too had been isolated in a special room, off the post partum area, because of the infection. I gave her a report, saying that Falecia was doing "better than could be expected," but stressing the fact that the odds were against her—and us. I didn't want Faye to get hurt either, and I tried to prepare her for what the odds said we should expect.

I called Carol at her home in Arkansas and told her about the birth. Then I called Patty and told her and asked her to tell our mutual friends, including John. I hoped he wouldn't be needing his station wagon any time soon. After I hung up, I called my parents and Mom answered. She reacted to the news realistically, but bluntly, talking about where we should bury Falecia. She suggested Faye's family cemetery. Somehow, I resented her pragmatism. It seemed morbid. It was okay for me to think of Falecia's death, but my own mother? And she should talk! She came into the world seventy years ago weighing three pounds. I didn't know whether she was premature or just a low birth weight baby, but she was small enough to fit in a shoe box. And she grew up to bear six healthy boys—the largest, twelve pounds, and the runt of the litter was eight pounds.

I went back to the room, and Faye and I talked until quite late. It was a long conversation about diverse topics. She said she felt guilty about having a preemie, and about working while she was pregnant. Could her working have caused the premature birth? (We later were told that was not a factor.) She talked about the insensitivity of a medical personnel that would put preemie women on the maternity floor within sight and sound of happy mothers, fathers, and grandparents who came in to gaily gawk at their new relation in the nursery. She told me about a nurse who had come in for some small service and asked the perfunctory question, "How much did your baby weigh?" The response to Faye's answer was a heartless but probably realistic, "Oh, Honey, she'll never make it."

The nurse didn't mean to be cruel. She just didn't know the situation. The hospital probably doesn't think of the mental anguish preemie mothers, or mothers who have miscarried, go through to be stuck in the maternity section. It is probably just convenient to put them there. Faye and I talked about whether we should have more children, whether we should adopt, and how we should face our present circumstances. Then I fell asleep on the floor beside her bed. I was exhausted, but for some strange reason she wasn't, and she had done all the work.

The next morning I got up and drove back home, showered, and went to my classes as ill-prepared as I could have been. Word had leaked out to my students, and they too wanted some news. I felt rather like a freak, and I almost resented their interest and concern for the "little freak" we had brought into the world. Such feelings made me feel guilty, but I asked myself, "Why should I feel guilty for perfectly natural feelings?" The hope of the world is held in every parent's heart, and every birth is nature's attempt to improve on the human race. How *should* one feel when the baby that was expected doesn't meet the expectations? It would take time for us to adjust to the reality of the situation.

Because of the infection, Faye would have to be isolated until it was cleared up. She wouldn't be able to see Falecia for a few days, and she was taking antibiotics by an IV. I suddenly realized that I was a go-between for her and her baby. I wondered how she felt, being without Falecia. I also wondered what effect her separation would have. I knew from my experience that if a cow is not allowed contact with its calf until several hours after birth, she would reject it, even when it tried to nurse. The cow would actually butt it away. Would humans be the same way? Was that why the nurse encouraged contact when I first saw Falecia in the ICN? I learned later that there is a higher rate of child abuse among preemies than among normal babies. Could the reason be that their delicate condition did not allow for a normal bonding process?

Monday night Faye was feeling good when I drove up to see her after my classes. I also went to see Falecia in the intensive care nursery, scrubbing up carefully. There was no change, except that she had a tiny IV in her arm to feed her a solution of glucose. She looked thinner, if that was possible. She had a teacup-sized hat pulled over her eyes, and her tiny body was bathed in an intense light. "Jaundice," the nurse said, and she explained that most preemies get it. The light was phototherapy to help break down the dead blood cells that Falecia's undeveloped liver could not take care of.

I thought of all the organs and body systems that were being forced to function almost four months ahead of time, and I wondered if they could ever hold up under the strain. "She's at 40 percent oxygen. That's a good sign, considering how undeveloped her lungs are," the nurse said. "The room air was 21 percent oxygen, and many preemies must have 80 percent or 90 percent oxygen. The X-rays of her lungs were good. The infection your wife had probably helped her," she said. I was puzzled. "The infection probably forced rapid development of the lungs—of a substance called surfactant, a film that coats the surface of the lungs so that some air is trapped and the lungs do not completely collapse between breaths. If the newborn infant doesn't have enough surfactant, it will usually die of hyaline membrane disease. We usually call it 'respiratory distress syndrome.' "

The nurse tried to make her point clearer. "You may have read that President Kennedy had a newborn child die while in office. His child died because of this condition."

Her comment was almost totally lost on me, as I watched the respirator breathe for the naked, red being in the bright light. I had seen squirrels that were bigger. I marveled that Faye's infection may have indeed been the very thing that gave Falecia life now. Her body and Faye's body both somehow knew that survival in the womb was impossible, and chemicals and hormones began preparing her for survival in the outside world. But for how long?

I looked up at the heart-rate monitor. The light and the sound pulsed and ticked away. The dial read 180 beats per minute. As I watched, the sounds became slower, and the dial read 160, 140, 120 and then it dropped below 100, and a harsh-sounding alarm went off. The dial continued to drop, reaching 80. The nurse flicked Falecia's foot with her finger, and immediately the ticks became faster and the reading went up. The raucous alarm was silenced. Falecia's heart had slowed; mine, it seemed, had stopped. I had experienced the first of her many "heart rate drops." What caused them?

They didn't really know. Stimulation, sometimes rather violent, such as a thump on the chest, would cause the heart rate to go back up. With some babies, the nurse said, it would go down forever. The baby's heart would just tire out.

Suddenly, there was another decrease in the frequency of the ticks, and I watched the dial start to drop again. Keep it up! Keep it going! I silently prayed, hoping that the power of my thinking would increase the frequency of the ticks. The dial dropped down to 120, 110, and just before it reached 100 and the alarm would have gone off, it began to rise again.

I rubbed Falecia's foot, a miniature no longer than the joint of my thumb. It was a mass of little red pricks. In fact, it looked as if someone had been using her heel for a pin cushion. "We have to have blood to check her gases—to see how much dissolved oxygen is in her blood. That way we know what to set the oxygen at. Too little oxygen, and she will have brain damage; too much and she will be blind," the nurse explained. My mind was boggled by all the things that *could* go wrong, by all the things going on, by the explanations, and by the machinery. I needed help.

The next day, I went to the place that had always provided everything I had ever needed when confronted with a difficult situation—the library. When I had needed to overhaul a tractor on my parents' farm, it was the library that had provided a book with a step-by-step process. The library always had provided me with information and had helped countless times before, but this time, there was nothing. I couldn't believe it. There was absolutely nothing about premature children. No information, no solace—nothing. We were in this thing alone, and we were blind.

I called Faye to tell her not only about the library failing us but also give her the latest news about the baby. (I found myself frequently using such impersonal terms—the *baby* or *it*, rather than Falecia. I wondered if I was protecting myself by trying not to admit that Falecia was a real person who was just tiny and undeveloped.) When Faye answered, she burst into tears. I thought the inevitable had happened. The baby had died while I was at home, and Faye had been given the news. I tried to wring information from her long distance, and between sobs, I learned that nothing was wrong. Faye was feeling well; she had received good reports on Falecia. We had had our first encounter with the post partum blues.

The post partum blues was explained in Dr. Spock's book, but the several paragraphs about premature babies were about how to feed them and how to care for them after they were home. If Falecia survived, that information wouldn't apply to us until she came home, bringing with her a huge hospital bill. I knew that our insurance would pay part of her bills, but there would still be a huge drain on the pocketbook that hardly anyone could afford, and certainly not a teacher. But I resolved to pass that bridge of bills when I got to it.

Faye finally got to see Falecia Thursday. Her baby was still active, and constantly flailing her arms and legs about so much that she had actually kicked the respirator tube above her head. Except rather than weighing a pound and a half, she had lost weight. She was now only 15 ounces. I thought how little that really was when I was doing some grocery shopping and bought a pound of margarine. My baby weighed the equivalent of about three and three-fourth sticks of margarine! I later learned that weight loss is normal the first several days.

Falecia was being fed through an IV. How they had threaded the tiny needle into the equally tiny vein in her arm, I'll never know. They had fed her a glucose solution for several days by an IV in her umbilical cord, but that method was now impossible. They had shaved the fine hair off her arm, and had begun the IV with TPN, or *total parenteral nutrition*. So she would not knock the needle out, the nurse had taken tissue paper, made tiny ropes of them, and tied her arms and legs down. I later learned that most babies have so much body fat that giving them an IV in the arm is next to impossible. The normal procedure is to thread the needle in a vein in the head where blood vessels are close to the skin. The sight of an IV in the head is rather shocking for parents if they are not aware that the needle is only in the skin. The sight of the shrunken, wire-ridden body, tied down under the heat lamp must have been more than Faye could bear, despite my preparation. She broke into tears.

My parents also got to see Falecia for the first time that day. Mom was still pessimistic, even more so after she had seen what she had imagined. She still was worried about a burial place. Faye's mother had seen the baby two days earlier, and although she had seen lots of shocking sights in her sixty-eight years—births, many deaths, even a murder—she wasn't prepared for the little wired robot in the heat crib. She nearly passed out.

A DOCTOR SPEAKS

17. What can I expect my premature baby to look like?

That will depend on how premature the baby is, but don't expect your child to look like the Gerber Baby. It is indeed a shocking thing for some people, being used to seeing full-developed babies, to see a scrawny, immature human being. In the case of a baby as small as Falecia, the medical profession is actually given the task of turning a fetus into a human being. That is why even a woman as experienced and hardened as Falecia's grandmother reacted as she did. Of course her reaction may have been influenced by the fact that she was related to the baby in question, but I have seen total strangers crying at the sight of premature children in an ICN. There are some people who will not even look at babies in an ICN because of their emotional reaction.

When you see a premature baby for the first time, the most obvious differences will be in size and weight, both of which will depend on gestational age. The lower the gestation age, the lower the weight and the smaller the size will be. Also, the baby will not be plump, but thin and spindly. Your baby's skin will be very thin and transparent. You will be able to see many of the baby's blood vessels because of the absence of the small layer of fat beneath the skin. You may also be able to see bones and muscles.

Your baby may also be very hairy. This very fine body hair, called lanugo, develops between the fifteenth and thirty-second week, so preemies often seem furry. But it will soon disappear, just like it does on babies still in the uterus. Your baby also may have little spots on the skin or nose, which are really immature sweat glands. Usually, they disappear in a few weeks.

Like a full-term baby, the preemie may have some or no hair on the head, depending on the individual. And like a full-term baby, he or she will have a "soft spot," the fontanel. This soft spot is where the bones of the skull are not completely grown together. You may sometimes see the baby's pulse there, but the soft spot is actually quite tough and can be touched. It will close at about one or two years of age.

Because muscles and nerves are not fully developed, preemies seem shaky or jittery when they move, and they lie stretched out like scrawny fledglings. As the baby grows, it will gain more muscle control and its movements will become less jerky.

I have found that many parents are concerned about their baby's belly button. This place on the baby's abdomen where the umbilical cord attached the baby to the mother is called the umbilicus. Like a full-term baby's, it must be cut at birth, but often a preemie is fed a solution or given drugs and medicine through an IV inserted into the umbilical blood vessel. The IV line that is used for preemies is actually not a needle at all, but rather a long plastic tube that is placed through the umbilicus into the larger artery in the abdomen. There is no way to predict what any baby's belly button will look like when it gets older, but preemies often have small hernias that close without requiring surgery or gadgets to hold pressure on the hernia.

Parents always seem to look at fingers, toes, and ears. The baby has had fingers and toes since twelve weeks after conception, but they are small and seem enlarged on the ends. Nails may be just tiny dots. The ears are made of cartilage, a tissue that doesn't fully develop until the final weeks of pregnancy. As a result, a preemie's ears seem like a soft, wrinkly skin, but they will become firm later.

The preemie can hear and see. The baby will be aware of monitor noises and voices, and some preemies seem to respond to the soothing voice of a parent. Bright colors and objects that are near are more easily seen, but it is not known for sure how good the eyesight of a preemie is. Some parents make a point of wearing the same, brightly colored clothing when they visit their child, of calling him or her by name in the same tone of voice, and even of wearing the same cologne or perfume so that the preemie learns to associate them with certain smells, tones, and colors. Preemies, like normal children, are taking in information from their world through their senses.

18. Will my premature baby exhibit different behavior from a full-term baby?

Behavior is a matter of development and maturity. We see that in children of different ages, and the same holds true for children who are younger than we are used to seeing. Since a mother may not have seen a preemie before, it is difficult for her to know exactly what behavior to expect. You must expect the reflexes and responses of a preemie to be different from a full-term baby. Here is what you may expect:

- Sucking—A baby's suck reflex is developed as early as twenty-six weeks on into the pregnancy. However, it is usually not strong enough for drinking until thirty-three weeks. Falecia, because of her extreme prematurity, had not yet developed the suck reflex.
- Swallowing—The swallow reflex develops early, but swallowing is very tiring for a preemie. The reflex is not well developed until about thirty-four weeks, and the baby must learn to coordinate swallowing with sucking and breathing.
- The Startle Reflex (also called The Moro Reflex)—This is the reflex that causes the baby to automatically flail its arms and cry. It is caused by a loud noise or sudden movement. Because preemies develop more slowly outside the womb than inside, this reflex may last for several months past the preemie's expected birth date.
- Crying—One of the things that amazes people who visit an ICN is the absence of crying. They expect that if there are twenty babies, at any one time half of them will be crying. In preemies, however, crying is seldom seen or heard. As the baby gets older, it will cry more, and louder.
- Grasping—The reflex to grasp is seen in the tiniest preemie. It may not be very strong, but it increases in strength as the baby gets older.
- Hiccups—Visitors in an ICN are often concerned by the spasms that violently rock a preemie's body, but these "spasms" are merely hiccups and actually seem to bother the baby very little. They are normal for all babies.
- Bowel Movements—Like all newborn infants, a preemie's first bowel movement is dark black/green "meconium" which consists of old hair, skin cells, and blood that has been swallowed during the early part of the pregnancy. These bowel movements will become more normal once feedings are started.

19. Are pre-term babies provided with special care at hospitals?

Almost all hospitals now set aside an area in their regular nurseries for their larger and healthier preemies. Very small or sick babies receive round-the-clock attention by nurses and "mother machines," as the special equipment is called. Such babies are placed in ICN's where specially trained nurses care for them under the supervision of neonatologists, doctors who specialize in treating newborns.

If a hospital is not equipped with an intensive care nursery, it may transfer the baby to a specialized center shortly after birth. Preterm babies are rushed to such centers, often by aircraft, so that they can receive the best care available, and so that their weight and condition can be carefully monitored.

20. How often is my premature baby weighed?

If your baby is very sick, or is burdened by a variety of monitors and machines, and if weighing is likely to cause even more stress, the infant is best left alone. Normally, however, babies in an ICN are weighed every day. Weight loss or gain will indicate how ill he or she is or how poorly he or she is doing.

Parents often become alarmed at the initial weight loss of their premature babies. Such a weight loss is normal, even among healthy, full-term babies. This initial weight loss is extra body fluid, and the low weight is reached four to twelve days after birth. The baby will regain its birth weight in one to three weeks, depending on the amount of prematurity and the severity and length of its illness.

Most ICN staff members encourage parents to be concerned about their baby's weight. Such concern gets you involved in a relationship with your baby. You should not hesitate to ask the ICN staff about your baby's weight. In addition, if you live a long distance from the intensive care unit, call and ask about your baby's weight. Many hospitals now have a toll-free number for parents to call to check on the progress of their child. Calling is one of those things you can do to establish a relationship with your child, despite the distance.

21. Grams do not mean a thing to me. Why don't doctors use pounds and ounces when talking about my baby?

Doctors use the metric system because it is an international system, and because they are trained to think in metric terms. For most people who are not used to the metric system, it is difficult to gain a concept of weight when it is expressed in grams.

Following is a conversion chart which you may find helpful.

WEIGHT CONVERSION CHART

POUNDS / OUNCES →	0	1	2	3	4	5	6	7	8	9	10	11	12	13	14	15
0	GRAMS	28	57	85	113	142	170	198	207	225	284	312	340	369	387	425
1	454	482	510	539	567	595	624	652	680	709	737	765	794	822	850	879
2	907	936	964	992	1021	1049	1097	1106	1134	1162	1191	1219	1247	1276	1309	1332
3	1361	1389	1418	1446	1474	1501	1531	1559	1588	1616	1644	1673	1701	1729	1758	1786
4	1814	1843	1871	1898	1928	1956	1984	2013	2041	2070	2098	2126	2155	2183	2211	2240
5	2268	2296	2325	2353	2382	2410	2438	2461	2495	2523	2552	2580	2608	2637	2665	2690
6	2722	2750	2778	2807	2835	2863	2892	2920	2948	2977	3005	3034	3062	3090	3119	3145
7	3175	3204	3232	3260	3289	3317	3343	3374	3402	3430	3459	3487	3516	3544	3572	3601
8	3629	3657	3686	3714	3742	3771	3799	3827	3856	3884	3912	3941	3969	3997	4025	4059
9	4082	4111	4139	4168	4196	4224	4253	4281	4309	4338	4366	4394	4423	4451	4479	4508
10	4536	4564	4593	4621	4640	4678	4706	4735	4763	4791	4820	4848	4876	4905	4933	4961

22. Does the life of my premature baby depend on technology?

To a great extent, yes. The machines do for the baby what the baby and its systems cannot yet do. Often technology tries to duplicate the environment in the womb so that growth and development can take place as rapidly as possible. For example, the developing baby is cushioned from shock and temperature changes by the fluid in the womb. Many hospitals now use tiny "water beds" for preemies. Warm and gently rocking, the heated incubator water beds simulate the floating environment of the mother's womb. It has been found that babies on water beds grow faster and experience fewer breathing and heart problems. Water beds also keep pressure off joints of preemies who have not yet developed adequate muscle and the protective layer of baby fat.

A study at Georgetown University Medical School showed premature infants kept on water beds gain as much as 25 percent more weight and had greater head growth than preemies on conventional mattresses. The study also showed that they could be handled more easily by the nurses, and they could be rolled from side to side. In addition, the babies would often curl up in the fetal position, something that they cannot do on conventional mattresses.

Technology provides what has been denied the baby as the result of its premature entry into the world, but it must be used by skilled technicians and loving and caring nurses, coupled with parental concern and visits, if the preemie is to thrive.

23. There are so many machines attached to my baby. Why and what are they for?

Parents who are unprepared for their first visit to the intensive care nursery may feel they are entering a world of science fiction. Unbelievably tiny babies lie in incubators amid bright lights, mechanical noises, and various life-support systems. Babies with breathing difficulties receive oxygen through hoods placed around their heads or plastic tubes inserted in their windpipes or noses. Those that suffer jaundice caused by immature liver function require special lights around the incubator. Very small or sick babies have their heart rates, breathing, and blood pressures continually monitored by machines that sound an alert to nursery staff at the first sign of trouble.

Babies may initially receive nourishment and medication intravenously; later, milk (even breast milk pumped from a mother who wishes to nurse) can be fed from a tube inserted into the baby's stomach through its mouth.

It's easy to understand that parents' first visits to their pre-term baby can be upsetting. The strange surroundings and obvious efficiency of the nursery staff may cause them to feel inadequate and uncomfortable.

The reaction of parents at the first sight of their preemie child on various life support systems can range from shock to awe to bewilderment. Remember, every parent expects to bring a normal, healthy, full-term baby into the world. When the circumstances are altered, and we find that the baby has not met our expectations because it is born early, sick, or deformed, there is a good deal of disappointment, and a great deal of adjustment is necessary.

The sight of a sick, tiny baby, wired for life is not the vision a parent had expected for what is often the first meeting with his or her child. But if the child is to survive and live to grow up normally, those machines and monitors are necessary. First, parents should recognize that these machines are divided into two categories. There are those machines that actually assist the baby in some aspect of his vital functions. Then there are machines or monitors that give the nurses and doctors instant readings of certain vital signs that allow them to better care for the infant.

In the category of machines that assist the baby is a device that actually helps the baby to breathe. Many infants do not have the muscle strength to take adequate amounts of air in when they breathe. As a result, many premature infants are attached to a breathing machine—a respirator or ventilator. This machine basically pushes small amounts of air into the baby's lungs to assist the baby's breathing. It is most often connected to a tube passed through the mouth or nose, between the vocal cords, and into the baby's main airway, called the trachea. These plastic tubes are called endotracheal, or E-T, tubes. This E-T tube also allows the nurses to draw mucus out of the baby's airway, preventing it from becoming clogged. The respirator is used on the babies who are the weakest and need the most help in breathing.

Babies who have more strength but still need small amounts of extra oxygen or pressure to help keep their lungs inflated are often on CPAP, pronounced "see pap." The initials stand for Continuous Positive Airway Pressure. Usually, the CPAP is applied to the infant with small nose prongs that slip into the baby's nostrils. Although you may think that the baby's nose is going to be forever stretched and that it will grow up with a "gorilla nose," long-term problems are uncommon. After the baby is off the CPAP, the nose will return to normal, and the breakdown of skin tissue at the nose will heal in a few days.

For babies who have no trouble breathing but who need increased oxygen, there is a device called an oxyhood. It is simply a hard, plastic bubble that fits over the baby's head as it lies in its crib. The plastic bubble provides a small, artificial atmosphere that contains just enough oxygen for your individual baby's needs.

The other category of machines is monitoring equipment, devices that allow the nurses to instantly read vital signs of the infant. This makes their job easier, and it also allows them to know the condition and state of certain important body functions, so that they can make changes instantly that can make the difference between life and death, and a normal or a brain-damaged infant.

One of these devices monitors heart rate. Many premature infants have multiple patches attached to their chest which pick up the faint electrical pulse each time the heart beats. The primary purpose of the heart monitor in these infants is to carefully observe the child's heart rate, because premature infants often develop episodes of bradycardia, or slow heart rate because of the immaturity of the heart's regulatory system, in addition to many other factors.

Oxygen monitors are attached to the respirator or to the plastic hood. These monitors determine the concentration of oxygen the premature infant is breathing and provide a readout of that concentration. Such monitors have a built-in alarm system that sounds if the concentration of oxygen gets too high or too low.

This monitoring is important, and the new technology will save even more babies in the future. Falecia owes her life to this kind of technology, and although she was tiny and ill-formed when she first came into the world, because of those "mother machines," she has life and an opportunity to develop into a normal, productive person.

24. What is the most critical system for the premature baby?

Because the human body is an interlocking system of systems, it is difficult to say any one system is more important than the others. Life depends on the working of all those systems. But if one is to pick the system that is most crucial to the survival of a premature baby, it would be the respiratory system. If a premature baby does not survive, death is usually caused by a failure in the respiratory system or complications in the other systems brought on by a poorly developed or functioning respiratory system.

The primary respiratory organs are the lungs. Also included in this system are the passageway between the nose and lungs, the ribs that protect the lungs, and the diaphragm, which serves as a pump to move air in and out of the lungs. A premature baby's respiratory system is forced to begin working before it is developed. Certain machines can take some of the burden off the baby, but even the techniques used to save the baby can cause stress.

For example, the pressure from a respirator required to inflate the baby's lungs may cause some scarring and damage to the lungs, even when low pressures are maintained. This damage is called bronchopulmonary dysplasia, which, although not identical, can be compared to emphysema in an older person. This scarring prevents the lungs from transferring oxygen from the air to the blood as efficiently as they should. As a result, the cells of the body become oxygen starved.

Another technique used to take a load off the premature baby's respiratory system is to give the baby more oxygen than is found in normal room air.

25. Are most premature babies given oxygen?

Yes, initially. Oxygen is the air that fires the fuel (food) of the body. Take away a fire's air, and it smothers and dies. Take away a person's oxygen, and he smothers and dies. The administration of oxygen to a sick baby or a premature baby in greater concentration than exists in ordinary air makes it easier for the baby to breathe and raises the oxygen level of the blood. Ordinary room air, at sea level, contains 21 percent oxygen. Giving the baby 30 percent, 50 percent, or even 100 percent oxygen, eases the stress placed on its immature body.

A baby's very life depends on the lungs. In the womb, the baby was provided oxygen via the placenta and the umbilical cord by its mother. Now that the baby is born, no matter how prematurely, it is forced to breathe on its own. If it is deprived of oxygen for more than four minutes, the baby will suffer irreparable brain damage. The brain has about fifteen billion cells and, as the nerve center of the body, regulates a vast number of its activities. These fifteen billion cells require lots of oxygen. Brain cells use oxygen at a much faster rate than do other cells of the body. That is why a baby's head is always so warm. The heat is caused by the rapid consumption of oxygen. Actually, about one-fifth of the oxygen absorbed in the lungs is used by the brain.

The lungs, which have about 300 million tiny air sacs, each with its cobweb of blood vessels, provide the oxygen to the brain and the other body organs. In the lungs, the red blood cells pass single file in the maze of blood vessels to pick up oxygen to carry to all parts of the body via the blood system. While in the lungs, the cells also discharge the waste product, carbon dioxide, which results from the body's consumption of oxygen.

26. How do they find out how much oxygen is actually being carried in the baby's blood?

By a blood gas test. A tiny amount of blood is taken from the baby, usually by pricking the heel or one of the umbilical vessels. Laboratory tests will show the amount of oxygen in the blood, and the level of oxygen administered to the baby can be increased or decreased as needed. The frequent testing requires blood transfusions because the infant's blood-producing organs are immature and cannot replace the blood that is required for the blood gas tests.

The frequency of the testing (often every hour or two) may seem cruel, and it may leave the baby with a scarred heel, but that is preferable to a scarred retina. Before the advent of such careful monitoring, up to 90 percent of surviving infants whose birth weights were below four pounds suffered total or partial blindness because of retrolental fibroplasia, a condition caused when high concentrations of oxygen damage the membrane of the eye's nerve endings or cause abnormal blood vessel growth on the retina. Now only about ten percent suffer any eye damage, and total blindness is rare. New techniques are constantly being developed that are more accurate and less traumatic to the infant. For example, a transcutaneous (through the skin) monitor which measures the oxygen in the child's blood stream was developed recently. Such a monitor has the advantage of showing nurses how efficiently the child's respiratory system is transferring and using the oxygen. This device is proving to be one of the most important technical advances in the field of neonatology. The device warms the skin to increase blood flow. Consequently, the TcPO2 (Transcutaneous oxygen) monitor may leave small red circles on the skin, but they quickly fade away.

Another new device actually measures one parameter of oxygen in the infant by use of a special light transmitting glass fiber built into the wall of a plastic catheter used in the umbilical artery. The two devices allow almost constant monitoring of the infant without blood loss for testing. However, at the present time, blood samples are still used, combined with the new devices, for standardization and closer monitoring.

27. Does the oxygen usually help?

Yes, if the lungs are mature enough, and if the infant can produce enough surfactant. Surfactant is a film that coats the surface of the lungs so that air is trapped and the lungs do not completely collapse between breaths. Normally, during the last few weeks of pregnancy, the fetus manufactures this substance in preparation for life outside the womb.

When the fetus leaves the womb before enough surfactant is produced, the result is hyaline membrane disease, often called "respiratory distress syndrome." This is what kills, directly or indirectly, most premature babies. The disease is rare in full-term infants, but about 10 percent of all premature infants may have it. Each year, up to 40,000 infants die from this disease.

If the infant has hyaline membrane disease when born, the condition may progress to death within a few hours. In milder cases, the symptoms reach a peak within three days. After that, gradual improvement is noticed. When recovery occurs, the outlook is generally good, although recurrent and prolonged lung infections are more common among survivors.

The longer the premature baby survives, the greater the chances of recovery. And although the disease is actually an oxygen deficiency disease, studies of babies receiving vigorous intensive care suggest that these infants don't have more mental disabilities than babies of similar weight and gestational age who did not have the disease.

28. If oxygen is good for the baby, isn't more better?

No. Too little oxygen can cause brain damage, but too much oxygen can result in eye and lung damage. Years ago, oxygen therapy babies were given 100 percent oxygen without any qualms. This actually damaged delicate blood vessels in the lungs and eyes and nerve endings in the eye. At that time as many as 90 percent of the infants on oxygen therapy were affected by retrolental fibroplasia. Because the level of oxygen is so critical, close oxygen monitoring, either through the skin or through blood gases tests, may be required every several hours. Because of this careful and frequent monitoring of oxygen, only about 10 percent of those babies who go on the respirator and oxygen suffer eye damage.

29. What kind of eye damage can result from too much oxygen?

The most common is retrolental fibroplasia. It occurs because the increased oxygen causes fragility of blood vessels in the eyes and a sudden growth of blood vessels in and around the retina, the small light-receiving screen on the back inner two-thirds of the eyeball. This blood vessel growth and breakage cause damage to the immature retina. Often the retina will detach from the back of the eyeball, causing vision problems and even total blindness. Even if it doesn't become detached, mild to severe scarring and distortion of the retina are likely.

Your pediatrician will have an ophthalmologist examine the

baby's eyes during and after the oxygen therapy to see how severe, if any, the damage is, and he will make suggestions for repair. When the doctor looks into the eye with a special instrument, he can easily see the location and the extent of the damage. There is no pain involved in this procedure, despite the fuss your baby may make. There has been much recent progress in surgery to repair retrolental fibroplasia damage.

This surgery, which is done under a microscope, is used only in some cases. First, the cornea and lens are removed. Then, with a tiny spatula, the scar tissue on the retina is scraped away. The retina is pushed back into place, and the lens and cornea are stitched in place. Although the child will always need glasses, this surgery prevents total blindness. But it must be done when the baby is six months to a year old, before the retina has fully matured and hardened.

If the retina does become detached, there is still the possibility of spontaneous reattachment, and often the abnormal growth of blood vessels regresses after the oxygen therapy is discontinued. If the retina does not reattach itself, one or more operations may be necessary to reattach it. A specialist, skilled in this treatment, uses a tiny point of very intense light, or in some cases, extreme cold, for a fraction of a second to create very tiny particles of scar tissue that "glue" the retina back to the inner surface of the eyeball.

Treatment is usually successful for a detached retina if it is done before the damage progresses too far. Your baby's ophthalmologist will keep you posted on progress and remedies.

30. Why is an incubator necessary for my premature baby?

Our word *incubator* comes from the Latin word meaning "to lie in or upon." A chicken incubates her eggs to hatch them. Likewise, an incubator is an artificially heated container for hatching eggs. If you think of your premature baby as not yet hatched, you can see why such an artificial environment is necessary.

A normal, full-term baby comes into the world with lots of baby fat, which is used to maintain body temperature. This fat serves as the baby's insulation and helps to keep the temperature of its body and internal organs at their best operating temperature and condition. A premature baby lacks this baby fat, however, and as a result can't maintain the correct body temperature. Consequently, the baby's temperature has to be artificially regulated with an incubator. You may have heard stories about premature babies born at a time when most births took place in the home and the intensive care nursery was unknown. Our pioneer ancestors had to improvise incubators, and there are stories of preemie babies being kept warm in the back of a wood cookstove, or with hot water bottles. Sometimes, the baby's crib was surrounded by quart fruit jars filled with hot water to keep it warm.

The modern incubator serves the same purpose, but it is slightly more sophisticated. It is basically an enclosed unit with a heater connected to a temperature probe, which is connected to the baby. When the baby's temperature drops below a certain level, the heater kicks on and warms up the baby's tiny room. Some babies are kept in open units because they require more care and it is easier for nurses and doctors to work on them unencumbered by a glass or plastic bubble. But the open unit operates much the same way. Its heater will kick on and maintain just the right temperature for the baby.

As infants grow older, they may tolerate brief periods of time out of their heat support systems (just as we can tolerate brief periods of time in a walk-in freezer), but they do require close watching. Gradually, as the premature baby gets older, gains weight, and adds to its insulation layer, it will be able to maintain its body temperature and will graduate from the incubator to a normal, open crib.

31. Why must I scrub up and wear a gown in order to see my child? These procedures make my visit seem forced and artificial.

The job of scrubbing hands and nails carefully and wearing an isolation gown at all times may seem awkward and cumbersome, but when you realize you may bring in germs that may infect your child and other babies in the ICN, you will remember to practice this ritual religiously.

Such procedures are essential in caring for premature infants because their immune system, the system that fights infections in the child, is, at best, poorly developed. Likewise, the signs and symptoms of infection are also poorly developed in a child. The premature infant, for example, may not run a fever with infection. Rather, its temperature may drop. Overwhelming infection in a premature infant, referred to as "sepsis," represents one of the more serious problems in caring for premature infants.

Good hand washing and isolation techniques may represent a cumbersome chore for the parents (and the nurses) of a premature infant, but they are some of the more critical procedures in an intensive care nursery. In fact, the scrubbing ritual may be good therapy for the parents. It certainly allows them to show their concern, and their ability to do something for their child.

32. The first time I saw my baby in the ICN, there was a needle in his head. Why?

Often it is necessary to feed sick babies intravenously, or through a hollow needle inserted in a vein. In normal, full-term babies, who have a nice thick layer of baby fat, it is next to impossible to find a vein and thread the needle in it. In such babies, the only place where the veins lie close to the surface of the skin is on the head, and so a head vein is used. Even in premature babies which lack the layer of fat, a head vein is often used.

It is a matter of necessity and convenience, and no harm results. But it can be a frightening sight if a parent is not prepared for it or does not know the reason for it.

33. Why are some of the babies in the ICN wearing diapers and others aren't?

An intensive care nursery is no place for an overly modest person. Mark Twain said that man was the only animal that blushes—or needs to. The lack of clothing may embarrass you, but it won't bother the babies. In fact, it is probably better for them, especially the younger ones. Falecia, for example, wore no clothes for the first two months of her life, and for good reason. Premature babies have very fragile, tender skin. The smallest amount of pressure will bruise or break it. Clothing would tend to worsen the condition of their skin, and certainly a premature baby doesn't need to be exposed to any more stress than necessary.

In addition, it is easier for the nurses and doctors to work with the babies. The reason nurses jokingly give to this kind of question, is, "It saves diapers."

Only the older, more mature preemies—who do not require as much close attention and whose skin is ready to face the rigors of the world—will be wearing diapers.

34. Will my premature baby boy be circumcised?

Only if you wish. You must sign an operative permit for this procedure, and most doctors would rather you wait until the child is much older and more stable. Premature infants do not tolerate stress of any kind, and technically unnecessary procedures like circumcisions are best delayed. If you are debating the decision, the Ad Hoc Task Force of The American Academy of Pediatrics has some findings and recommendations that may be of interest. Among their findings:

- There is no convincing scientific evidence to substantiate the assertion that circumcision reduces the incidence of cancer of the prostate.
- There is evidence that carcinoma (cancer) of the penis can be prevented by neonatal circumcision; there is also evidence that optimal hygiene confers as much or nearly as much, protection.
- Circumcision should *not* be performed on newborn infants who are premature or seriously ill or who have bleeding problems or any congenital anomaly (especially hypospadias). It is also recommended that it not be performed in the delivery room immediately after birth but delayed until the infant is at least twelve to twenty-four hours old.
- Of course, cultural and religious factors, as well as medical ones, play a part; and the final decision regarding circumcision is the parents and should be based on true informed consent.

35. Will I be allowed to take a picture of my preemie?

Most ICN's will not object to your taking a picture of your baby, but you should ask the staff members first. It is better to take a picture under existing light conditions if possible. Since an ICN is well lighted, you won't need high-speed film to get excellent pictures.

Falecia, for example, will have some absolutely amazing pictures to marvel and wonder at when she gets older because her father frequently took pictures.

If you don't have a sophisticated camera or high-speed film, even a flash picture should not be objected to. Babies in the intensive care nursery live in a world of twenty-four-hour light and constant beeps, clicks, noise, and voices.

36. My initial reaction when I saw my premature baby was, "Why didn't the doctor let it die?" That was a month ago. Now I feel guilty. Is that normal?

Yes, this is normal, and entirely to be expected. The child born was not the ideal child you had expected. As a protective mechanism, you refused to become too attached to the child so that you would not suffer as much grief and pain if the child did not survive. When the child did survive, you felt guilty for those earlier, perfectly natural feelings.

One of the problems to cope with in caring for premature infants, both from the parents' standpoint and the neonatal intensive care unit staff's standpoint, is in the area of the critically ill, damaged, or obviously dying child. Most physicians have had experiences with infants whose future and survival were very much in doubt, but who survived without significant damage. On the other hand, infants who had relatively few problems can subsequently have fairly significant damage. One of the biggest problems that the intensive care units have at present is trying to predict which child will survive without damage and which child should have less aggressive care. Miracles do happen in an ICN. A baby everyone expects to die, for some unknown reason, will pull through. On the other hand, a baby who had minor problems will take a turn for the worse, and die or be damaged.

Many parents feel guilty when relatives and friends encounter them after their premature baby has been discharged from the intensive care unit—especially if the child has had some physical damage—with a look on their face that reads, "It would have been better if that infant would have died." My reaction is always, better for whom—you, who are reminded of the problems in the world by looking at the baby? And who are they to decide, when they don't really know the history of the child? Alexander Pope has a maxim, "Whatever is, is right." We may not agree with that, but we must live by the maxim, whatever is, we must accept.

Besides, one's standards of what is acceptable usually change when one has such a child. A parent cares for a child, even a normal one, with a certain lack of certainty in the outcome of his or her life. We all know physically handicapped young adults who are full of life, and we read in the newspaper every day of physically beautiful young adults who have committed suicide. Most of us would take the former for our child any day, rather than the latter.

37. Is it possible to have my premature baby baptized?

Baptisms are seldom a problem. You may send a priest or minister from the church of your choice to baptize your baby. Often, even one of the nurses of the ICN will baptize your baby for you.

38. Is there anything that I can do as a parent that will help the bonding between my baby and me?

Bonding is the term given to the emotional attachment that grows between parents and children, especially between mother and child. Falecia's father worried about the lack of contact he and his wife had with their preemie. He thought that a lack of contact might result in their rejecting their baby, much like he had seen cows reject their young after having been denied contact immediately after birth.

Although humans cannot be equated exactly with animals, it is true that preemies are rejected more than full-term babies. Some are abandoned by their parents in the ICN. Preemies are more subject to child abuse than full-term babies.

But to answer your question, yes, there are things you can do to help the bonding between you and your baby. Try to have as much contact as possible with your premature baby. Spend as much time as possible at the ICN. If ICN policies permit it, become involved in the care of your baby. Apply lotion, wash and change the infant, and help with the feeding—anything that involves you with your preemie will help the bonding process. Make clothes for your child, even if he or she can't yet wear them. Make a tiny toy or buy one for its incubator room. Ask the nurses questions about care and development. They will be glad to get you involved.

If your child is in a regional ICN and you can not make frequent trips for visits, make frequent calls to check on the progress of your preemie. Some ICN's have a toll-free hotline for parental calls. Take pictures of your preemie when you do get to visit, and when you are home, involve yourself in activities that include the long distance baby—making clothing or toys, planning the nursery, keeping a diary for the baby, or keeping a detailed babybook.

Parental involvement, even at long distance, will increase the parent-child bond. Parental and professional awareness of bonding is producing dramatic changes in hospital nurseries, and even in the intensive care nursery. It used to be that the fear of infection converted the ICN into a fortress where sick and premature babies were kept in strict isolation. But things are changing. Parents are encouraged to visit the ICN to cuddle, stroke, feed, and care for their premature child. If your pediatrician or the ICN doesn't allow such visits, without having adequate reasons for the policy, demand time so that you can have contact with your baby. The visits benefit both you and your baby. Many neonatologists now believe that the physical contacts of touching, stroking, and rocking help the baby's breathing and physical development.

Most doctors and ICN's encourage parent-premature baby contact. Nurses will make a special effort to get reluctant parents to touch their premature baby. Some nurses and hospitals, aware of bonding problems, have letters written to parents in the baby's name, explaining progress and preemie problems from a preemie's viewpoint and signed with his footprint. Some ICN's take pictures and send to parents. Many nurses leave personal notes from the preemie's viewpoint on the incubator for parents to read when they visit.

Some hospitals have special programs to educate and reassure parents of premature children. And there are even some hospitals that have experimented with nesting—an arrangement that allows the mother to stay with the premature baby in a private room several days before the baby is discharged. Such an arrangement allows mothers, who often feel inadequate about caring for their child, to become comfortable, and it allows the ICN staff an opportunity to teach the mother any special care techniques the baby may require.

39. What stresses can parents expect to encounter after the birth of a pre-term baby?

Parents may experience strong, conflicting emotions after the birth of their child. Feelings of fear about their baby's condition or about their ability to care for the child are alternately replaced by feelings of hope and pride. Disappointment may occur when hopes for a chubby, cuddly baby are dashed by the reality of the small and skinny premature infant, whose head may appear too big for his body and whose body is covered with fine hair and delicate skin. Parents sometimes feel angry, wondering why their baby was born prematurely, or they may blame themselves and experience intense guilt. Then there are moments of gratitude and joy that wash away such feelings.

Studies have shown that mothers of pre-term babies often experience erratic mood changes—feelings of depression and worry interchanging with happiness and relief—for months after delivery. Leaving her baby in the hospital for weeks or months after returning home adds to a mother's concern. Hospital visits may be difficult to manage. The visit may be a greater problem if the baby is being treated at a special center at some distance from home. Although telephone contact with the nursery is helpful, it is not as reassuring as being with the baby.

Fathers have their share of problems, too. Aside from dealing with their own worries, they are the prime source of comfort and support for their wives, who are often physically and emotionally drained. During the first critical days of the baby's life, a father may become closely involved with the infant's condition and care. His initial concern for his wife's welfare turns to the baby, and he may have more contact with the medical staff than she does during the first few days. If the mother is incapacitated or is in another hospital, she may feel left out or jealous. As time goes by, and the mother becomes actively involved with the baby, the father may feel left out and jealous, particularly if he feels his needs are being neglected.

Emotional ups and downs are normal responses to stress, and

parents may find coping easier if they can communicate their feelings and respond to each other with sympathy and understanding. The need for emotional support continues after the baby is brought home. There is joy and relief, but there are also ongoing pressures and worries. Because pre-term babies are biologically younger and less-developed than full-term babies, they require more attention and more feedings. In addition to other stresses, research indicates that parents find the crying of pre-term babies more irritating than that of full-term babies.

40. Will the premature child affect our marriage?

Very likely so. Every action has a reaction. The birth of a premature child is a crisis in the life of a parent, and during a time of crisis, parents often retreat from reality and regress. They may even find themselves behaving like children. In rapid succession, they may become demanding, overly critical, or angry. Some parents withdraw, becoming depressed and refusing to visit the child.

As the child's condition will vary in the intensive care nursery, so will your response as parents. Certainly an unresponsive, sick infant, who is passive and burdened by monitors and machines, will not successfully engage his parents, nor will you as parents derive any pleasure from him in the way that you would from a normal baby.

If you are the baby's mother, you may lose confidence in yourself as a woman and mother. You will probably question your ability to care for and nurse the baby because it requires specialized nursing care. If you are the baby's father, you may secretly resent your wife for not having the "perfect" child, and you may retaliate by being moody, angry, or critical. By being aware of the typical responses, you may be better able to deal with this traumatic incident in your lives.

chapter three

HOW TO BE PARENTS FROM A DISTANCE

A PARENT SPEAKS

As parents, we had decided we would do all we could do to make Falecia "normal." We bought her a toy—a tiny, soft, yellow bootie—but beside her in the Isolette it was almost as big as her head. We had learned from the nurses that preemies do better if they have such attention paid to them. Parents who believe will buy a doll that is bigger than their 2 lb. baby, and put it in their child's Isolette. And a funny thing often happens. The 2 lb. baby with the doll in the Isolette gets better and grows bigger. If it worked with two-pounders, perhaps it would work with Falecia and bring her back up to a pound, and then two pounds. A tiny kewpie doll, about the size of the bootie, soon joined Falecia in the incubator.

Although we didn't have a child at home to prove it, we were parents, and we decided to carry on as if things were normal, hoping that by doing so they would become normal. Faye had resolved that she was going to breast feed the baby when it was born. The sudden change of events didn't change her resolve, even though several nurses told her that it would be months and months before Falecia could nurse—if she survived—and that the various formulas would be more than adequate. Faye didn't listen, and with the encouragement of Dr. Griesemer and several of the nurses, got an electric breast pump and began pumping and freezing milk, saving several bottles of colostrum—the milk that is first produced after birth.

It was a good thing that she did. Falecia did not tolerate the TPN at all, and although Dr. Griesemer had doubts about her digestive system being able to handle milk, there would be nothing to lose by trying. A tiny tube—called a gavage tube—was threaded down Falecia's throat and into her stomach. The milk was pumped down the tube, a few drops a minute, because her stomach would not have been large enough to handle even a half a teaspoon at one time. Amazingly, Falecia's undeveloped digestive system could handle it, and she took to the breast milk like a duckling takes to water. Out came the IV, and off came the ropes that tied her down. Falecia could now kick to her heart's content.

Friday, Faye would get to come home. I came up for her after my last class. I brought my camera. I wanted some pictures. The baby was almost a week old and we had no pictures—except an in-womb polaroid snapshot of the ultrasound picture taken before Faye's cervix sewing.

I got permission to take pictures, and I scrubbed carefully, but I didn't remove my ring. Instead, I scrubbed carefully around and under it—a single white gold band. The camera was a 35mm, only a year old, a replacement I had bought after losing my old faithful on a float trip on the Buffalo River. In Falecia's isolated room, I bent over her heat crib. Below me was the constantly moving baby, who had a respirator that breathed for her eight times a minute, a tube down her stomach to feed her, a heart monitor patch on with a wire running to the alarm system, and another patch that measured the dissolved oxygen in the blood vessels just below the surface of the skin. Falecia may have looked like a robot, wired for life, but she was mine. I kissed her inch-long foot—a definite "no no" I'm certain—but no nurses were around to see.

I snapped several pictures, and then I removed my wedding ring. It easily slipped over her hand and up to her shoulder. I took several pictures. My ring just as easily slipped over her leg, except that it was difficult to make the 90° turn at her ankle. It slid up past her knee. I marveled at how small, but perfect Falecia was. There were tiny dots for fingernails and toenails. Her eyes were open, but there were no pupils yet visible. It was obvious that she saw forms because she would move her eyes toward movement. The bright heat lamp, however, caused her to keep them closed most of the time. Much of the time, she wore a black "skull cap" that covered her eyes, to protect them from the special light that was part of her phototherapy for jaundice.

Falecia seemed to have no vocal cords. When I had watched her heel pricked for her blood gas test, she had wrinkled up her face and had turned redder, but made no sound. She was crying without a voice. There was no way to show pain or displeasure, except by wrinkling her face.

I realized I was a witness to a sight seldom seen by most parents: The development of their baby before it is born. Falecia had been due in the middle of August, a Leo, but had instead been born at the end of April, a Taurus, the sign of the bull. She needed the strength of one, I thought. I really shouldn't think of her being almost a week old. She wasn't even born yet. That attitude would be important, because that way I wouldn't think of her being behind, of not developing normally. I would have to calculate her progress, from the time she should have been born.

Falecia's genitals consisted of an overly large clitoris with no labia, or fat pads, on either side. There was no fat on her at all. She didn't have a baby's chubby cheeks. I could see every vein, every artery beneath the surface of her skin, and I could see them pulse with each beat of her tiny heart. It was the lack of a protective insulating layer body fat that caused Falecia not to be able to maintain her body temperature, hence the heat lamp,which though it dried her skin, was absolutely necessary for her survival.

Since her birth, I had heard all sorts of stories about premature babies born before such modern marvels. My grandmother had kept my mother warm by putting a hot water bottle in her shoebox crib. Mamma Luce, who lived up the street from us, had kept her premature first child warm by actually putting her in the open oven of her wood cookstove. And another woman, who worked on campus in the printing department, had lain in a crib ringed by fruit jars of hot water. Her parents changed the water in every other one every half hour. These primitive incubators were not the best, but at least they were better than certain death.

I don't know what it is, but most people are interested in preemies. Perhaps it is concern to give and show support, perhaps it is just curiosity, perhaps it is the freakishness of these babies. It seemed as if Falecia generated an interested (and often to me, interesting) following. My students often inquired about her, especially the agriculture majors. My student secretaries asked for progress reports. Faye's students called or got information from their friends and parents. Our church regularly asked for reports, until the church secretary put up a picture of Falecia, along with adequate space to record weight gains. We received cards from friends, acquaintances, and total strangers. Nurses in other areas of the hospital often checked on her. In the ICN, she became something of a celebrity, because she was the smallest baby to have survived so long.

I realized the interest of others several weeks after her birth when I was outside the ICN waiting for the reports to be finished and the shift to change so that I could go in. A grandmotherly looking, black cleaning lady was peering into the nursery, trying to catch a glimpse of the interior in the crack of the drawn shades. I asked her if she had a grandchild in the ICN.

"No, suh," she replied. "I just checks that little baby in the back room when I cleans B wing. I always says prayer for the little thing. Can't hurt nothing, and it could even help."

If prayer has any power other than the power of positive thinking, Falecia had a multitude pulling for her—various church groups, neighbors, students, and ourselves. Friends and even total strangers, would remark that she was being remembered.

The Branson Cafe and The Shack, two of our local cafes that served the town rather than the tourists, and which served as an auxiliary office for me—a place where I could escape office phone calls and interruptions, be free to grade papers, read, or write—soon became additional places where I couldn't get work done. People would come over to my table and ask about Falecia, tell me that she was remembered in their prayers, tell me about a friend (or neighbor, or relative) who had had a premature baby and who was now a strapping youngster and doing well in school. They always told the success stories, I noticed. What about the failures? The ones who died or grew up blind or brain damaged?

But like these people, Faye and I also focused on the positive. The Friday Faye came home, we settled down for the long, hopeful wait. It was a grind that grated the nerves raw. But Faye's coming home didn't settle our lives. For the third Sunday in a row, it was back to the hospital. This time it was for a retained placenta. After Falecia was born, all of the afterbirth had not been expelled, and so Faye had to go back for a D & C. I wondered, was there no end to our problems and complications?

Faye's doctor was out of town, and so one of his colleagues performed the operation. I sat in the waiting room, along with my brother who lives in Springfield. He is a perfectionist, the kind of person who delights in intricate inlays in guns he builds, and he spent all the time straightening the pictures in the waiting room. My mother-in-law was also there; she worked on her sewing. I just sat, wondering if there could be any more problems in our lives, wondering about Faye, about Falecia, and about my classes.

The operation didn't take long, but Faye had lost a good deal of blood, both before and during the operation. She had to be given two pints. Falecia, who had to have her heel pricked every two hours to check the amount of dissolved oxygen in her blood, had also had several transfusions. In her case, often a teaspoonful was all she needed, but each time, the hospital counted the transfusion as a complete unit. I had given blood once already to replace an earlier transfusion, and because of the time limit the Red Cross imposed between donations, I would be in debt several gallons by the end of the month. I didn't dare think of how much money I would owe.

I knew that our group insurance would cover the hospital bill, but only for seventy days. But there were various other bills—lab tests done outside the hospital, the pediatrician's fee, various specialists' fees. These people would also be demanding payment.

I had learned from Dr. Griesemer that most states have programs to cover "high risk" pregnancies and births, and the social worker at Cox Medical Center had visited Faye soon after the birth. She encouraged bonding to a child that wasn't up to birth expectations, but also explained about this high-risk program. In fact, the social worker had filed the necessary forms for us. About a week later, I received a letter stating that Falecia did not meet the medical criteria for the program. I was amazed. If she couldn't be considered high risk material, what baby would meet their standards?

Since I had a meeting in the state capital the next week, I decided to delay any investigation into the matter until that time. In Jefferson City, after my talk on unusual place names in the Ozarks to the state meeting of librarians, I called the director of social services, and inquired about the medical criteria.

I learned that there was weight criteria for premature babies. Funding could be given only for babies with a birth weight of between 800 and 2000 grams. Falecia had weighed 700 grams. I was stunned. What did this mean? Did legislators and the doctors who had given advice in drafting the legislation believe that no attempt should be made to save the life of a baby that weighed less than 800 grams? Did they think these babies, because of their size and lack of development, should be quietly allowed to die in a sink in the delivery room? Hadn't medical technology and pediatric science made advances that justified new criteria?

I did some thinking on the subject, and then it dawned on me.

It was a matter of politics. Some of the babies I had seen die in the ICN could have lived. Neonatal intensive care units have to compete for money and staff, which is really another way of saying dollars, since personnel costs money, with other more visible, more vocal voices demanding tax money. ICN's even must compete within the hospital system with other, better-known, and more visible aspects of hospital care, such as those units for heart attack victims. Parents who use the ICN are temporary, episodic users of that health care system. Their baby gets well and they take it home, or it dies. In either case, they no longer have contact with the hospital. Such parents don't pressure hospital governing boards or state officials to improve neonatal care facilities. But a heart attack victim knows full well he may need that facility in the future, and so the pressure is on to fund and continually upgrade those kinds of hospital facilities. It just wasn't fair.

I hotly fired off a letter about the weight policy to my state legislator that night, and I personally refiled the application under another of the various medical criteria—premature rupture of the amniotic sack. Along with the application, I had to file last year's 1040 income tax form. Now that looked bad because a financial need had to be demonstrated. And last year, on paper, we looked very good. There was my salary as a college teacher. There was Faye's salary as a teacher. Although Missouri ranks in the lower one quarter among states for salaries paid to teachers, and southwest Missouri is the lowest paying area of the state, our combined incomes and lack of a family gave us a comfortable existence. Making our financial situation look even better, we had withdrawn $6000 late in December from our life insurance/annuity that we had used to consolidate some debts and have a sum available for the rather unexpected expenses of even a normal birth. What was irritating, despite the fact we were paying the insurance loan of $6000 back, was that it had to be counted as income, and so we had wound up paying $600 in extra income tax just before Falecia was born.

So in December last year, it looked good on paper; in May this year—it wasn't nearly as good as it looked in reality. Faye was no longer teaching. We had the mountains of unexpected bills. There was only my salary. As I had expected, a week after application, I received a letter informing me that we did not meet the financial criteria for the program. So that avenue was blocked. Another path out of the financial maze would have to be found.

In the meantime, there were other things to worry about. I had finals and summer classes to prepare for, and term papers to grade. We called the ICN each morning and evening for a report, and tried to make the long drive to Springfield every day to see Falecia. We would usually go after my last class of the day, see Falecia (we had a fifteen minute visiting limit, but it wasn't strictly enforced), then go to a movie or out to dinner, return to the hospital for another short visit, and then make the long drive home again. After I finished grading papers or preparing for the next day's classes, it was often past 2 A.M.

Falecia was gaining weight on the breast milk, and by the second week in May, she was almost back up to her birth weight of one and a half pounds. Rather than being fed drop by drop, she was fed two cubic centimeters every hour, then four cc's every two hours, and gradually her milk ration was increased. Dr. Griesemer knew the number of calories in a gram of breast milk, and a simple computation based on body weight told him how much milk was needed for her metabolism. Falecia was being fed as much as possible, and her weight gain was the proof of the pudding. Anyone that disputes the virtues of breast milk should look at some spectacular results. I didn't think the few ounces she gained was all that spectacular, until a friend in the college's Agriculture Department commented that he could get rich if his hogs would gain that much that fast. I wasn't used to the hospital's metric system, and it was a bit difficult for me to visualize grams and cubic centimeters. I decided to check, to put things in familiar terms. I filled the hypodermic needle I had used to vaccinate our cat to the two cc mark. Then I forced it out. It exactly filled the half-teaspoon on Faye's set of measuring spoons.

On Mother's Day, we had arranged to meet my parents at the home of Faye's parents. I had dug up two waho trees, rather rare native species, sometimes called "hearts bursting with passion" because of their peculiar red, heart-shaped seed pods, which burst open in the fall. Both mothers were avid gardeners and plant collectors. The talk at that Mother's Day noon meal, however, was not about plants, gardens, or the weather, but about Faye being a mother now and Falecia. We had to bring them up to date on her progress, and they were proud of her increase in weight. We explained to them about her heart rate drops, and we told them that Dr. Griesemer had prescribed aminophylline—a heart stimulant, to decrease their severity and frequency. We couldn't explain what it was that really caused them because it really isn't known for certain.

We also explained to them that we were fortunate Falecia had not developed any heart problems, at least not yet. When the baby is in the womb, its blood does not flow through the lungs to any great degree. It gets all its food and oxygen from its mother's blood. But as soon as it is born, a vessel closes, forcing the blood to go through the lungs to pick up oxygen. In preemies, this vessel does not always close properly, and heart surgery is often necessary to permanently close the vessel. As far as we knew, despite Falecia's small size and the lack of development of her lungs and heart, this vessel had closed and sealed. There was no murmur.

After we returned home, I presented Faye with her very first Mother's Day card and gift. Neither of us had expected last year that we would ever be celebrating Mother's Day. We hadn't even expected to be celebrating this Mother's Day even after we found out that Faye was pregnant. It was a strange situation being parents and non-parents at the same time, and Falecia's mother adjusted well to the situation. I wouldn't have wanted any other mother for my baby girl.

It was already quite late, but since an intensive care nursery never closes, we called for our nightly report. It was not what we expected. Falecia had had her worst day ever. She had had numerous heart rate drops. In fact, her heart had almost stopped a number of times, despite the stimulant. And she did not respond well to body stimulation to bring her heart rate back up. It was taking her longer and longer to get the beats up to their normal range. She seemed to be tiring out. The nurse was concerned. That was evident by her voice. There was not the usual guarded but optimistic tone that we had become used to. She was preparing us for the worst. And so Faye cried herself to sleep that night, with her first Mother's Day card under her pillow.

A DOCTOR SPEAKS

41. My baby is in the intensive care nursery. It almost seems like I'm not a parent. Why do I feel that way? Will my feelings hurt the child later on?

It is only natural that you have such feelings. After all, you have brought a child into the world, but that child has been taken away from you. You have willingly allowed those who can better care for your child under these extreme circumstances to take control. You are a parent, but you don't have the normal duties of a parent. It is indeed a frustrating position to be in.

First, recognize that the separation is necessary if the infant is to survive. It is in the best interests of the child that the separation exists, and all parents want what is best for their child. Second, remember that the separation is temporary. As soon as the child does not require special care, you will be able to assume more responsibility. Thirdly, it is important to minimize this separation by visiting your baby in the intensive care nursery as often as possible in the weeks or months before the baby is well enough to bring home. Doctors now know that the sooner babies and parents make contact with each other, the better it is for both. Even the sick and tiny babies seem to benefit from the stimulation of human contact. Preterm babies appear to gain weight more readily when they are touched, talked to, held, and rocked. Also, parents who spend more time with their babies in the hospital usually are more comfortable caring for them at home.

Questions about parents' feelings toward their premature infants are now taken very seriously. Studies have shown that the rate of child abuse is higher among premature babies than among fullterm babies. This higher rate may be caused by the higher percentage of young, ill-prepared parents who have such babies. They may have difficulty accepting the trials and tribulations of parenthood, especially parenthood that demands their accepting a child that isn't their "dream baby." It may be caused by the lack of bonding that is caused by the isolation of the child from the parents.

The fact that you are an intelligent person, and are aware of the problems that will develop in your relationship, will make those problems more easily solved. If you feel you don't have enough contact with your baby, and are worried because you don't, it may be comforting to realize that families who adopt children usually make excellent parents without the benefit of early bonding.

Nurses, doctors, and hospitals are becoming increasingly aware of bonding problems, and they are making changes that allow a stronger and more natural bond to develop between parents and premature babies. In the past, parents were not allowed into an ICN; they literally gave up their baby until the hospital staff decided the infant was stable enough for them to become parents again. Now most ICN's encourage and even insist on parental visits and participation in the care of their premature child, especially as the child gets older and stronger and no longer requires respiratory support and incubator care.

42. How is a premature baby fed?

Most problems with premature babies are caused by the fact that their body systems are forced to function weeks or even months ahead of schedule. This is true of the preemie's digestive system. Since conception, the baby has been fed with nutrients drawn from its mother. When it is forced out of "the hatchery" earlier than the average forty-weeks gestation period, its stomach is still immature and will not absorb foods readily.

Initially, most premature infants are fed either through an umbilical artery catheter, which is a plastic tube inserted through one of the vessels in the umbilicus, or navel. Or the baby is fed through a vein in its hand or scalp. A solution with sodium, potassium, and carbohydrates is infused through these plastic tubes until the baby is old enough to take feedings.

Some premature babies are mature enough that they have a well-developed suck reflex, and they can be fed formula or breast milk by bottles with a nipple. If the baby does not have a well-developed suck reflex, and if it can tolerate formula or breast milk, a gavage (sounds like *garage*) tube, or feeding tube, is passed through the infant's mouth into the stomach, and food is slowly poured directly into the stomach.

Sometimes this gavage tube is kept in the baby to avoid stimulating certain important nerves that control the heart. Usually it is inserted with each feeding, and although it looks like a tricky business, nurses do it quickly and easily. The possibility of the tube entering the baby's lungs or poking a hole in the baby's stomach is slim.

43. Which is better for a premature baby, formula or breast milk?

A very strong case can be made for breast milk, and most pediatricians will say it is better than formula. Breast milk is the product of millions of years of evolution and development, and it isn't likely to be replaced or duplicated. It has been called the ideal milk for infants because it has all the necessary food elements in the right proportions. It digests easily and rapidly, and babies are less constipated and have fewer attacks of diarrhea. An excellent book that discusses the advantages of breast milk and breast-feeding over formula is *A Doctor Discusses Breast-feeding* by Marie Pichel Warner (Chicago, Budlong Press, 1970).

44. Does breast milk have any advantages over formula?

One of the dangers to premature babies is sepsis, or overwhelming infection. A mother's first milk, called colostrum, includes substances that help protect the baby against disease. Colostrum provides the baby with certain antibodies, which are natural substances that protect the body against a specific disease or infection. In a sense, it is a kind of vaccine the mother can provide the baby to help combat the various organisms that can cause infections.

Another advantage of breast milk over formula is not actually found in the milk itself but in the act of breast-feeding the premature baby after it is able to come home. Feeding the infant at the breast gives it a feeling of warmth and security that is important for its well-being. More importantly, it provides a better and stronger bond between the mother and child, which may have been weakened or not developed at all because baby and mother were separated for so long. Breast-feeding may help a mother accept her baby, especially if it was damaged by its prematurity. However, some mothers can't breast-feed, and holding the baby while giving him his bottle, and giving him lots of love and attention while he is eating, may be just as effective in the bonding process.

45. I want to give my premature baby breast milk. What should I do?

First, make your desires known to your doctor and pediatrician. Get help and advice from the intensive care nursery staff. If the baby is fed your breast milk while in the ICN, whether by bottle or gavage tube, you will not have to wait until your baby comes home for him to become used to your milk.

You will have to hand express your milk every three or four hours during the time the baby is in the ICN. You can use a breast pump, a small, hand-operated device that removes milk from the breast by suction. Or, better yet, the ICN may have an electric breast pump you may use. If not, you may be able to rent one. The electric breast pump consists of a motor and pump which is connected by plastic tubing to a glass or plastic cone which fits over the breast. The electric pump provides the suction, and as the milk is withdrawn, it flows into an attached bottle.

If you have difficulty getting an electric breast pump, contact La Leche League for help and advice. The nursing staff at the ICN or your doctor should be able to give you the local chapter's address and phone. You can always contact La Leche League International, 9616 Minneapolis Avenue, Franklin Park, Ill., 60131 for information about nursing and breast milk or the location of its many local branches and chapters.

The milk you express can be refrigerated or frozen until the premature baby is able to use it. And more importantly, you will keep your flow of milk going until the baby is able to come home.

46. I was going to breast-feed my premature baby, but it was simply impossible, and now I feel guilty. Why?

It often happens that a mother can't breast-feed her premature baby, no matter how strongly she may desire to. First, the baby may be so premature that it is not able to nurse. If it is able to nurse, the mother may not be able to be at the ICN at its feedings. The trauma of having a preemie, and all the problems and worries such an experience entails, may dry up the mother's milk supply.

As a mother, you may desire to give part of yourself, to try to become involved with your baby, despite the fact that others are caring for it. Such desires and efforts are admirable and commendable because they foster a bond between mother and child. But when circumstances conspire to prevent you from breast-feeding your child, you shouldn't worry about it.

In addition, the intense desire to breast-feed may be a psychological compensation for the guilt feelings that a mother may have for bearing a premature baby. There is no reason a mother should have such feelings in most cases of prematurity, but many mothers do have them. This worry alone would be enough to dry up your milk supply. Face facts. If you can't breast-feed your baby, you can't. Don't worry about it, or feel guilty about it. There are various formulas that your baby will thrive on.

47. I was going to have my premature baby fed breast milk, but my milk dried up. Will my baby have to switch to formula?

Not necessarily. Some large hospitals have their own milk banks. Others buy breast milk from commercial agencies that collect breast milk from healthy mothers who are nursing their own babies. The milk is sterilized and then frozen, a procedure that replaces the old time wet nurses who substituted for mothers who were unable or unwilling to nurse. Ask the ICN staff about breast milk, or contact the La Leche League. They will be glad to help you.

Although most pediatricians believe breast milk is a better food than formula, many also believe formulas provide good nutrition. Most infants, unlike Falecia, will tolerate and thrive on formula, and formula does have some advantages.

48. What advantages does formula have over breast milk?

Formula is easier to obtain and store at the intensive care nursery than breast milk. It is often less trouble for the ICN staff and the mother, factors that many parents may consider. In addition, because of changing social and cultural patterns, many mothers have employment outside the home that does not give them the flexibility they need for breast-feeding. Some mothers may be physically unable to nurse their babies. Although the trend seems to be changing in the other direction, studies have shown that more than 80 percent of all babies, and even a higher percentage of preemies, are fed with formula.

Other reasons mothers give for not nursing are the limitations on the mother's or parents' social activities, a fear of failure at breast-feeding, the fear of weight gain or loss of attractiveness because of changed breast structure, and even the belief that breast-feeding is not socially acceptable.

For some parents, formulas may be the preferred, or only, method of feeding. With a better understanding of milk chemistry and food processing, industry has developed milk formulas and soy-based formulas that offer unprecedented versatility and freedom to mothers. These include special formula preparations designed specifically for premature infants.

In addition, you may consider a combination of both breast and formula feeding, a practice which is becoming very common. A combination of formula and breast-feeding gives the baby the advantages of the mother's antibodies, but allows the mother more flexibility with her social and business schedule.

49. My premature baby has jaundice. Is that common?

Yes, jaundice is common even among normal, healthy full-term babies. In fact, approximately 50 percent of all full-term babies become slightly jaundiced during their first week of life.

In the case of preemies, the incidence is much higher—about 97 percent. Falecia, you may recall, had jaundice. The more premature a baby, the more likely it will require treatment for jaundice.

50. What is jaundice?

Our word for this condition is derived from the French word *jaune*, which means *yellow*. The condition results when a yellow bile pigment carried in the blood, called bilirubin, is deposited in the skin, the mucus membranes, and the whites of the eye. It causes the characteristic yellow color.

51. What is bilirubin?

Bilirubin (pronounced Billy Rubin) is the subject of many ICN jokes about unusual baby names, like, "Do you know Billy Rubin's real name? Yes, William Rubin." Actually, bilirubin is the end product of the breakdown of used red blood cells, the cells that have the oxygen-carrying red pigment called hemoglobin. Usually these red blood cells break down slowly and consistently as they age and become worn-out. The bilirubin that is released is carried in the blood to the liver. In the liver, it is processed so that it can be excreted from the body via the intestine. If for some reason the liver does not do its job adequately, bilirubin accumulates in the blood and is deposited in the skin and membranes. In the case of preemies, the liver does not do its job simply because it is immature.

52. Is jaundice dangerous?

The jaundice color itself is not dangerous. However, the bilirubin which causes the jaundice can cause brain damage if it is allowed to reach excessively high levels. Fortunately, bilirubin is photoactive, and exposure to certain wavelengths of light will break the bilirubin down and allow it to be excreted. This is why you may see your premature baby—or even a full-term baby—wearing a black skull cap to protect his eyes as he is exposed to light. The bilirubin count is determined by taking a blood sample measuring the actual concentration in the baby's blood. A bilirubin level of 1 is considered normal. At a level of 3, there would be a slight not noticeable yellow or jaundiced appearance. Most infants reach levels of 5 to 7, which is considered normal. Bilirubin is currently considered dangerous at a level of 20.

Premature infants do not tolerate as high a level of bilirubin as full-term infants. In premature babies under stress, a doctor will seldom allow the bilirubin count to go much beyond the level of 10 before he or she intervenes.

53. Do premature babies often have heart problems?

Preemies often have heart problems, but they usually are not as serious as the phrase sounds. If the baby has a noncongenital heart problem, it is usually with the patent ductus, an opening between the aorta and the pulmonary artery. In an unborn baby, this is a principal conduit of circulation. It allows blood to circulate without passing through the lungs, which do not function in a fetus. The patent ductus is supposed to close at birth, or a few days afterward. In many preemies, it fails to do so. In the past, surgery was often required to shut the patent ductus. Now indomethacin, a drug used to treat arthritis, is being used to chemically close the ductus. When the ductus fails to close because of simple prematurity, indomethacin has helped in 75 percent of the cases. Other drugs are currently being tested, and perhaps some day one will be found that will make surgical closing of the ductus unnecessary.

There are numerous other heart problems. An infant may have, for example, a VSD, or *ventricular septal defect*. This is a hole between the two lower chambers of the heart, a problem which may resolve without requiring medical or surgical treatment. Remember, though, heart problems that were fatal a few years ago often can be cured today, and prospects for preemies with heart problems are improving all the time.

chapter four

"THE WORST"
IS NEVER
THE WORST

A PARENT SPEAKS

It was the worst night I think either of us had ever spent. There was no sleep until our minds exhausted themselves repeating questions that had no answers: Why had she done so well up to now? Why had she improved, gained weight, gotten bigger, if it was only to get our hopes up and then dash them? Why didn't the heart stimulant work? Why should it be her heart that gave up and just tired out rather than something else? Was the fact that it was her heart somehow symbolic?

The next day we made the long drive to Springfield. When we arrived at the ICN, we found that Falecia had improved considerably. She had had fewer heart rate drops,and she had been moved out of her isolation room. It was a remarkable departure from what we expected. She was out with the big babies—the preemies who weighed 3 and 4 lbs, and even more. It would have been enough to give her an inferiority complex. Although Falecia now weighed 1 lb. 8 oz., she seemed small next to the three-pounder on her left and the four-pounder on her right. And that night, a 12-pounder, a real thumper, was brought in. He wasn't premature of course, but was having lung problems. But the next time we came, he was gone. Death is always nearby in an intensive care nursery.

Prematurity is responsible for three out of four infant deaths, and in our trips to see Falecia, there were always moments when we wondered if life, that fragile bubble we all grasp, would be gone for her. Falecia, like all premature babies, was subject to episodes of apnea, when she would seem to forget to breathe. During these episodes, her heart rate would, of course, go down. A simple reminder, a jiggle on the foot, would start her breathing again. Other times, it would take more vigorous action, like a thump on the chest with the forefinger. Still, that might not be enough, and she would have to be "ambu'ed," to have oxygen forced into her lungs with a balloon-like device.

It was decided that the feeding tube might be irritating the vagus nerve and causing Falecia's frequent heart rate drops. It had been kept in place all the time to prevent excessive stimulation of the nerve which controlled the heart, lungs, and diaphragm. But when it was removed, there was no substantial improvement.

The respirator had started to cause some scarring of her lungs, so she was put on a *continuous positive airway pressure* device, called a CPAP for short. It also kept Falecia's lungs expanded, but the doctor hoped it would not irritate or scar her lungs as much. A cap with two prongs was fitted in her nostrils, with a salve between the two to prevent irritation and to provide an airtight seal. It had the oxygen tube attached to it. The cap came only in two sizes, large and small. The small one stretched Falecia's nose to the extent that when it was not in place, she looked like a tiny gorilla. I wondered if her nose would ever return to normal, but the nurses assured me that it would.

It was at this time that Falecia's vocal chords became developed enough for her to make noises. With the removal at each feeding of the gavage tube, she could now cry, but despite all the painful equipment that burdened her, the frequent pricks for blood gas test, I never saw her cry. Her tiny Taurus body braved all, and she lived up to the meaning of her name—felicity or tranquility. Through it all, she remained aware, but calm and tranquil.

Falecia had always been an active baby, moving her pipestem legs and arms about so that her monitor wires and tubes had to be carefully pinned out of her way. This characteristic had always pleased me, because I knew that "crib death," Sudden Infant Death Syndrome (SIDS), is more likely to happen to premature infants and babies who are not active or who do not display strong reflex actions. Falecia had been a sharp contrast to babies who lay quietly, passively in the ICN, almost seeming to be dead, except for the breathing done by a respirator. Perhaps SIDS was a worry we could put aside. At least it was one we wouldn't think about now.

We were now beginning to feel totally comfortable around Falecia, touching her and handling her, although she was still confined to her heat crib. I began to get to know the nurses better, and I felt no qualms at all about asking questions. I had always told my students that ignorance was reserved for those who don't ask questions, and in this new world of medical technology, neonatology, and pediatrics, I was a student—a first grader. Besides, since the library couldn't provide information, who else could I turn to? Certainly not our pediatrician. It wasn't that Dr. Griesemer couldn't or wouldn't answer our questions. He was simply too busy. (I could now appreciate complaints from my students who say they can't catch me in my office.) I did catch him long enough at his office to tell him the problem about the lack of information. He provided me with a number of medical and pediatric articles about specific concerns. They were informative, but they also contained much that I didn't understand because of my lack of medical training and even more that didn't interest me as a parent. They were written for doctors, not the parents of preemies. And so the next time I saw him, I suggested this book.

In the meantime, I became more aware of the other people around me in the ICN. I watched other parents, all of whom were younger than we were. There was a 13-year-old visiting her premature baby—her second one. There was a high school drop-out, a girl of about sixteen, who had a skull and crossbones tattooed on her arm, and beneath it, I detected needle marks. There was a father who drove sixty miles after cutting stave bolts all day, just to see his child. He had never gotten past the eighth grade. Most of the parents were young, they were often poor, but they were all human and concerned about their babies and the situation they found themselves in. Like me, they had no information to help explain their plight, to tell them what to expect.

One evening I watched as a horrified father saw his baby in the ICN for the first time. An IV had been started, and the needle sticking in his son's head caused his suntanned face to turn as white as the cabinets in the ICN. There was no reason that each of us had to be pioneers traveling a path no other could follow. There was no reason we shouldn't have had some help to explain the strange and fearful, to give us some hope or at least facts. Perhaps the lack of information was why some parents came less and less frequently. Perhaps that was why some parents never came at all. And perhaps that was why preemies are more subject to rejection and child abuse.

Faye had decided that if she couldn't be a mother to her child, she would make Falecia's surrogate mothers—the nurses—perform their best. It wasn't that they weren't good. I was amazed at their concern, their love for strangers' babies. They would pat them, talk to them, rock them, cuddle them, and give them everything their absent parents couldn't. I marvelled at how these nurse-mothers looked the part—loving and kindly. They seemed like "setting" hens with a flock of chicks, and the portly, red-haired head nurse, with her mother hen concern, seemed almost like the big Rhode Island Red we used to mother our mail order chicks with when I was growing up.

Faye thought that if she showed interest and concern, it would make the nurses more interested in Falecia, and make them better mothers. I don't know if it worked or not, but Falecia certainly got the attention from the nursing staff. One nurse made a tiny pacifier to help strengthen Falecia's sucking action. Another always taped a pink ribbon in Falecia's hair. Someone knitted a pair of teenie booties (the smallest pair one could buy would have looked like box cars ôn Falecia's feet). And although she couldn't have any of them, friends had given Falecia enough stuffed animals to populate a small zoo. And there were dresses galore—all, of course, far too large, but there was the hope of all that some day they would just fit.

The end of the semester arrived, and the summer-like Sunday after finals was graduation, a grand affair held in the fieldhouse. It was attended by parents and relatives, who watched as the new graduates and their teachers, in full academic regalia, marched to Sir Edward Elgar's familiar music to sit through the usual unheeded, unheard commencement speaker. Faye and I planned to celebrate the end of the semester by spending the afternoon after graduation at the lake house of a friend. I was to pick her up as soon as the whole hot ceremony was over.

When I arrived home, Faye told me that the ward clerk at the ICN had called, the first time the hospital had ever called, to report a change in Falecia's condition. She had had twenty heart rate drops already that day, many of them so bad that she had to be "bagged," or have oxygen forced into her lungs. We cancelled our part in the festivities, and although we knew it would not help Falecia in the least, we made the drive to Springfield. On the way up to Cox Medical Center, Faye told me she had been visited that afternoon by the Swopes, a young couple from a neighboring town who also had a premature child, and who had heard about Falecia. They had told Faye that compared to the problems their son had had, Falecia's setbacks seemed mild. First, his lungs had collapsed, and he had to be operated on. A heart murmur had to be fixed. The hospital in Kansas City, where very serious preemies from Cox were transferred, had called them three times, telling them to expect his death.

They had driven the snowy, winding roads out of the Ozark Mountains in winter to make the four-hour drive to Kansas City, wondering if their son would still be alive when they got there. He was one of the "success" stories.

Charlotte Swope had been there when Faye received the call from Springfield. I was thankful that they had been there to provide the support and help that I couldn't have provided, even if I had been there. There is so much that such parents, who have experienced the trials, tribulations, fears, and frustrations of being the parents of a preemie, can provide to new parents—information and comfort that no doctor or nurse can duplicate. In fact, some large cities have support groups for preemie parents. But in areas that don't, there is almost always a contact that provides parent-to-parent communication to help one deal with the situation.

As we drove, I thought of all the other babies I had seen in the ICN who had problems we and Falecia did not have to worry about. There was the baby who had been born not only prematurely but with joint deformities. Indications were that he was also retarded. He died. I wondered if his death was a blessing for his parents and for society. He would have been a million dollar baby, because of the care required in the ICN and because he would have been in an institution all his life. And what about the hydrocephalus baby, who had a tiny body with an adult-sized head, deformed and ridged like some creation of a science fiction movie? The child would always be retarded. We had not had any such serious problems. Falecia had always seemed normal, except that she was small. Up until now, she had done well. Were all our hopes to be dashed by her tiny heart, worn-out by her struggle to survive?

During the drive Faye and I were mostly silent, each of us lost in our thoughts. The quietness was broken only by traffic noises and a sniffle or two from Faye. When we got to the hospital, things had changed dramatically. Falecia had had no heart rate drops since they had called. She was quiet, resting well, and her heart seemed stronger. One of the nurses joked that this was just her way of getting us to come up and see her. It was a nice line, but we would have laughed at anything.

Dr. Griesemer was quite concerned because Falecia's apnea and associated heart rate drops were frequent and so severe. In fact, he said, some of them were more like seizures than typical heart rate drops. He explained that seizures were not uncommon among premature infants, and the smaller the baby, the greater the chances they would occur. Such activity, which may actually be called a tiny stroke, was caused by immature blood vessels in the brain breaking. Often, he explained, the baby would simply "grow out" of these seizures, but sometimes they were so serious and severe that the child would be affected for life, physically or mentally. There were certain medications that decreased the frequency of such seizures and lessened their severity. Dr. Griesemer prescribed a tiny amount of phenobarbital once a day.

After that episode, Falecia's apnea and associated heart rate drops gradually decreased in number and severity. Each time we would call the ICN, a morning and evening ritual, there were always two questions we would ask: "How much does she weigh?" and, "Has she had any heart rate drops?" With each passing day, her weight went up, and her heart rate drops went down. And the really good sign to me was that as her body weight increased her dosage of medication stayed the same. She seemed to be growing out of them.

Falecia also graduated from the CPAP to the oxyhood—a rigid, clear plastic "space helmet" that fitted over her head as she lay in the heat crib. Attached to it was a hose that provided the correct humidity and oxygen. It was her own special atmosphere, her life-support system.

The change to the oxyhood gave Falecia's nose a rest from the CPAP. The pressure of the CPAP, despite the salve that helped provide the seal, had stretched her nose and started breaking down the skin, leaving Falecia with a large scab. It looked as if she had taken a hard left to the nose, bloodying it and flattening it. But in a few days, her nose rounded out again, and the skin healed.

What was nice about the oxyhood was the freedom it gave Falecia and us. She was no longer confined to a rigid position on her bed. And our contact with her, which had been limited to touching, patting, and applying lotion to her dried skin, was increased. We were thrilled the evening we came and found the note taped to her crib, "Parents may hold." It was quite a procedure. A little hospital gown was put on Falecia. She was wrapped in a blanket, and then the oxyhood was removed and a little green mask was put on her, held in place by a piece of elastic. The oxygen line was then transferred from the oxyhood to the mask. I don't know if she enjoyed her new freedom, but we certainly did.

By now, Falecia was the senior citizen in the ICN. Other babies had graduated and been sent home, and the serious cases had been transferred to Kansas City or Columbia, or had died. Falecia received the attention and respect that should come with age. By now, she was a month and a half old, and she would have been six and a half to seven months along if she had not been born. She was filling out, getting plumper, although we were bothered by the fact that she had developed a long, narrow head. Her skin was getting better, especially when she was transferred to an Isolette—a large heat, humidity and oxygen-controlled plastic bubble that encompassed her entire body. Off came the oxyhood. I asked why she hadn't always been in one, and the answer I received was that so much must be done to care for such tiny babies that they must be exposed so the nurses and doctors can easily work on them.

Now that we could handle Falecia more, we began noticing new things about her. We noticed a birthmark, a tiny red streak on her left shoulder that we had mistaken earlier for a small scratch caused either by her own fingernails or a nurse. It was hardly noticeable, not at all like the large burgundy birthmark I had on my own arm. My mother, bless her soul, still insists that the reason I have the mark is that she was frightened by a fire in the barn while she was pregnant with me, and she still blames herself for not noticing it earlier than she did. She discovered it six hours after I was born, and by that time the afterbirth had been buried in the garden. She still insists that the application of the afterbirth to the birthmark would have drawn the color out. I didn't believe such old wives' tales, but I was amazed that many people did.

The same evening we noticed the birthmark, we noticed that her other shoulder, and especially her neck, was covered by a large yellowish-greenish patch—a very large bruise. We asked about it, and Daylene, her nurse for the night, shrugged off the question. Faye continued to press her about it, and finally she asked Daylene point blank. "It's a bruise caused by taking blood." "But why have they taken blood from her?" we asked. Daylene turned white, then a bright red. She explained that Dr. Griesemer wanted to run a genetic test. He was concerned about Falecia's genitals. There was some doubt in his mind that Falecia was a girl, or at least a normal girl.

How is one to react to such news? And should it have come from the nurse? Should the doctor have explained the test, or avoided parental anxiety by keeping it secret? It would take at least two weeks to grow the blood cells, "explode" them, and stain them to study the genetic and chromosomal material. Should he wait until after the test so as not to cause adverse worry?

Ever since Falecia had been born, there had been little change in her genitals. She still had, in comparison with the rest of her body, a large clitoris. In fact, it looked much like a small penis. And as yet, no labia had developed. She was slowly adding fat pads on her cheeks and elsewhere on her body, but not there. It is no wonder that her doctor and some of the nurses were beginning to wonder. Faye's reaction to Daylene's stammering explanation was to turn white—and then burst into tears. Mine was mute shock. I had wondered about the lack of change in Falecia, especially when one could easily compare her to other preemies in the ICN. Thoughts of sexual organ abnormality had flitted through my mind, but I had never seriously considered the possibility of genetic abnormality.

Debbie, the senior nurse on that shift, took both of us out of the ICN. The other nurses were looking at us; they all probably knew what had been kept from us. They had received the information in the report and update when they had come on their shift. They knew that we had found out. I momentarily hated them for keeping us in ignorance about our own child. Later, I wondered if I would have done the same thing if I were in their position. It wouldn't be easy to tell parents their child may be sexually or genetically abnormal, especially when lab tests had not yet proven it. What if the tests came back OK? You would have worried parents needlessly for two or more weeks.

In the nurses' locker room near the ICN, Debbie explained what was involved in the lab test, how it would be done, and what it would prove. I knew what they would be testing for because I had read widely about genetic abnormalities shortly after Falecia had been born. My mind wanted to block out what Debbie was saying, and so I lay on the bench and looked around the room. Blue uniforms were sprawled in open lockers, and street clothing was hung neatly. There was the smell of used shoes, old socks and sweat, but it was not as strong as a men's locker room. In addition, there was a faint undercurrent of a different odor, a combination of perfume and medicine. I wondered why my mind was taking all that in. I was very aware of it when usually I wouldn't have been. Perhaps it was a protective mechanism to block out unpleasant news or information.

Debbie left us to sort out our emotions. I lay on the bench, looking at the overhead light fixture. I remember thinking that it didn't look very clean. It was not at all sanitary in comparison with the areas that the patients normally saw. I comforted Faye, telling her I didn't think there was anything to worry about. I assured her that the reason the test was being run was simply because they wanted to be sure, and they were running the test now because they knew our insurance would soon be up. It only paid for seventy days of care. I told her that I was not really worried, because there was no evidence of the ridged, scrotum skin that is so readily apparent in male babies, no matter how premature they may be. I told her all these things, trying to make her feel better, trying to stop her from worrying. But I hadn't convinced myself.

From my college biology classes and from my recent reading, I knew that every normal person has two sex chromosomes in each body cell. A person with two X chromosomes (XX) is female. There is also a Y chromosome, and a person with the XY combination is male. But that was the normal person. The test would show several things. It would show whether Falecia had Down's Syndrome, often called mongolism because of the somewhat Oriental features such babies have. This congenital condition is more frequently found in children borne by women over thirty-five. Faye was thirty-five. I wasn't much concerned about Down's Syndrome, however, because Falecia didn't have the fold of skin at the inner corners of her eyes or the short fingers that are typical of such children.

The test would also show whether she had Turner's Syndrome, a disorder in females in which growth and sexual development are retarded. The arms and necks of such people are slightly deformed, and a person with Turner's Syndrome appears to be female, but has only a single sex chromosome in each cell—one X chromosome instead of the XX of the normal female. As a result of the single X chromosome, no ovaries develop in a person with Turner's Syndrome. There was also Klinefelter's Syndrome to be concerned about, but this congenital disorder is found in an apparently male person who has an extra X chromosome in each cell, making him an XXY instead of the normal XY. These men never develop testes, and they lack some secondary male sex characteristics, such as facial and body hair. I wasn't much concerned, as I didn't think Falecia was actually male.

There existed the possibility, however, that Falecia could be a hermaphrodite, a person whose body contains the tissue of both female ovaries and male testicles. The genitals of such a person may be either male or female, or a combination of the two. But true hermaphroditism is very rare, so rare that I would almost be willing to bet my life on those odds.

Although the genetic test wouldn't show it, there is a condition known as pseudohermaphroditism, or false hermaphroditism. This condition results from a response to the production of sex hormones. Such a person develops the secondary sexual characteristics of the opposite sex; a woman may have a beard and the deep voice of a man, for example.

I thought of Falecia with her thick, dark body hair and wondered whether she could have this condition. But all babies have such body hair during some stage of development, and they usually lose it before they are born. Falecia wasn't scheduled to be born until the middle of August.

Perhaps her unusual genitals were the result of the lack of adequate sex hormones. Was it possible that there had not been the necessary chemical trigger that caused the necessary sex hormone to be released and start (or retard) development of sexual characteristics? The normal person produces both male and female hormones in various proportions. Perhaps, because of her prematurity, her little body was not yet hormonally balanced. Only time, and the results of the test, would tell. In the meantime, we would have to just wait and worry.

A DOCTOR SPEAKS

54. My baby's sex organs do not look normal. Is she a sexual freak?

Not likely. Remember, you are used to seeing the sexual organs of a full-term baby. The sexual organs of a premature baby are not going to be fully developed.

In the case of a premature boy, the penis may be very small, and it may be difficult to see the foreskin over it. In addition, the testicles may not yet have descended from the body into the scrotum.

In the case of a premature girl, the clitoris may seem very large, and she may not have labia, the fat pads on either side of the clitoris. This may look very different from what you expect, and you may wonder if the baby really is a girl. However, console yourself. It is very normal for her to look like this at this stage of her development, and the sex organs will continue to develop as she matures.

55. My doctor said he was going to run a genetic test on my premature baby. Why?

Abnormalities in sexual development are very rare in all babies, including preemies. In Falecia's case the development of her external genitalia were felt to be unusual even for premature infants in her weight and gestation group. Both for the reassurance of the family and the staff, an early, definitive test to establish chromosomal sex is helpful. Unfortunately, the results can take days or even weeks to arrive and the unavoidable delay can be frustrating and difficult to handle optimally from all vantage points. Fortunately, Falecia was all girl, all 46XX of her!

The development of sexual organs in a premature baby will mimic the development of a baby who is born full-term. Consequently, the genitalia of premature infants may look smaller or somewhat different from what parents are familiar with in full-term infants. Sometimes the genitalia are so premature that the doctors will run a genetic test to check the chromosome count or the genes in the baby to determine the sex, or to see if the baby has certain genetic deformities, such as Down's Syndrome, Turner's Syndrome, or Klinefelter's Syndrome.

The development of sexual organs does not present a very serious problem in premature infants, but can cause concern. If you are worried, ask your doctor. However, most infants will develop normally, although many premature boys will have inguinal hernias that will require surgical repair later. The inguinal area is in the groin, particularly the abdominal wall near where the thigh joins the trunk of the body. Under strain, the groin area sometimes weakens, and the intestine pushes out. The operation to correct the weakness of the muscles is, as a rule, quite simple.

56. My premature baby has been in the ICN for almost two months and is developing a long, narrow head. Will this condition be permanent?

The long, narrow "preemie head" is commonly noticed in the ICN and will correct itself without any medical assistance. The shape of the infant's head is determined by a number of factors—the growth of the brain, the pressure of the womb before birth and the crib after the baby's delivery, and the pull of muscles on the baby's scalp.

Because the head is no longer supported in the fluid in the womb, an environment that is relatively weightless, it must be subjected to the pressures of its bed. Nurses in the ICN let the baby lie with its head turned to one side or the other. It is more comfortable and safer for the baby. If the baby spits up while a nurse is working with another baby across the room, it will not strangle on its own regurgitated fluids.

"Preemie head" is not dangerous. After the baby can better support the weight of its own head, and after you have it home and allow it to lie in other positions, the condition will disappear, and a normal, rounded head will develop.

57. Are premature babies more likely to die of crib death than full-term babies?

We know that SIDS infants are more likely to be premature, or at least small, to have young mothers, to come from poorer families or families that smoke cigarettes, and to fare poorly right after birth. Most premature babies fall into at least several of these categories. However, studies and statistics are inconclusive. Even the exact cause of crib death is uncertain.

SIDS claims an estimated 10,000 babies a year in the U.S., and most deaths involve infants two to four months old. Very few deaths occur in babies more than six months old. After the age of two, SIDS is unlikely. Research into SIDS is continuing. Specific differences have been found in the behavior of siblings of SIDS victims and siblings of infants who do not die during infancy. SIDS siblings have been found to be less mature in their reaction to visual stimuli. They smile less often; they take longer to tune out environmental noise during sleep; they are more irritable, and less consolable. They also have been found to be less adept at defensive maneuvers, such as using their hands to remove an obstruction that partially blocked their breathing. Most premature babies have these same characteristics.

There are many theories about the cause of SIDS. Recent research has even suggested that it may be caused by an allergic reaction to substances that irritate the throat and lungs. Any substance that irritates the child's airway may be a culprit. This may be why the incidence of SIDS among children exposed to cigarette smoke in the home is much higher than in children whose parents do not smoke. However, nothing is known conclusively.

Parents often feel somehow responsible when their child dies suddenly and unexpectedly. The feelings of guilt, loss, and concern may persist for a long time and cause immeasurable unhappiness, but your baby's pediatrician will investigate a death in which SIDS is suspected and provide an explanation and information, as well as comfort.

"Near miss" infants—those who have stopped breathing and needed external stimulation to restart respiration—are of interest because of shared characteristics with SIDS babies and preemies. Near miss episodes, which usually occur as the infant sleeps, causing the baby to turn blue and limp, are similar to the "heart rate drops" preemies often have. Full term infants who survive a "near miss" are considered to be at high risk for SIDS, as are premature infants, and both are sometimes put on home monitors that alert the parents if the child stops breathing. These record the infant's breathing, and sound an alarm if it stops. Costing more than $1,000, they are expensive and may be disruptive to the baby and the household, but these monitors can be lifesaving for those rare babies who doctors believe may need them.

Although no one yet knows why, the death rate from SIDS is declining. It was one in every 350 babies five years ago; today the estimate is one in every 500. In some states, notably Massachusetts, it is less than one baby in a thousand.

58. I fully expect my premature child to die, and I hate myself for having those expectations. Are my thoughts normal?

Your feelings are not only normal but, in the case of an extremely ill or extremely premature child, even helpful to you. You are preparing yourself for the inevitable. A dying child naturally evokes emotions of guilt, grief, and anger in parents. As a parent, you may feel guilty, thinking that somehow you caused the prematurity, but as I mentioned earlier, there are many causes, and most of them are beyond a parent's control.

Your feelings of grief on the expected death of the child are certainly normal. Death, including our own, is destined to remain among life's certainties. You are being realistic; you are not giving up hope. Just as the causes of the prematurity were probably beyond your control, so is maintaining life in that fragile, undeveloped body. There is no reason or cause to blame yourself. So much depends on the baby, on doctors, and on technology. There is nothing you can do except wait and anticipate.

The anticipatory grief that you feel is, in actuality, good for you. It allows you to expend your grief over a period of time. Although it may seem little consolation to a grieving person at the time, it is better for the individual in the long run. The responses of parents who lose children varies. The response to a stillbirth is likely to be less intense than the response to the death of a child who has lived a day, or to one that has lived precariously for two months in an ICN. Affectional bonding begins before a mother has physical contact with her baby and begins giving it care. Both contact and care increase this bonding, and although the mothers of most premature infants get little of this contact and care of the baby, they do establish an emotional bond with the baby, which increases the grief level. The longer the preemie survives, the more emotional capital a parent has invested in that child, and the more the parent will grieve.

Parents who do *not* have this anticipatory grief, and fail to face facts until the actual death forces them to face facts, have intense and longer periods of grief. In addition, they are more likely to suffer from confusion, guilt, severe depression, and "scapegoating."

Scapegoating is the opposite of self-blame. In the frustration following the death, the parent puts the blame on a spouse, other children, or, most often in the case of preemies, on the doctor or the nurses in the ICN. So your anticipatory grief should not be smothered. It is an aspect of your life situation that is normal, natural, and desirable.

59. If my premature child dies, what sort of emotional reactions can I expect in myself?

Modern pediatric medicine has made many advances. Today we have neonatologists who know far more than the old general practitioner could ever hope to know about newborns. These neonatologists have far better equipment, and their success rate in saving increasingly smaller preemies has increased, but tragedies have not been overcome. Certain tragedies are still found in the ICN, just as they were with the general practitioner or the midwife, and they will always be with us. The loss of a baby is one of those tragedies.

As a pediatrician, I, like many doctors, must sometimes be the purveyor of bad news. We employ hushed tones, as if such a method will somehow minimize the mutilation. But it doesn't. Whether the physician shakes his head, whispers, or shouts, the tragedy is still the same. That tragedy results in grief, one of the most common of human emotions. Yet it is one that most of us hesitate to even think about. When we are confronted with the grief of others, we feel awkward, and don't know what to say or do. When we do experience it ourselves, we seem helpless to accept and master it. We have no resources to meet it, and we use all kinds of defense mechanisms to avoid dealing with it.

Your initial reaction will be an emotional numbness. The British theologian C.S. Lewis said the initial reaction felt like being mildly drunk or having a concussion. Emotionally, you may expect the physical symptoms common to psychological incidents, such as pain or fear. You will have butterflies in your stomach, palpitations in your heart, and coldness and sweating at the same time.

Often the tragedy of the death of a preemie results in anger on the part of parents. Because they have no control over the situation, they often feel angry at those they believe to have control—doctors or nurses in the ICN. Just as often, parents are angry at the dead child, a reaction they feel uncomfortable with. It is a natural and instinctive reaction to pain. We strike back. It is much like kicking the chair that you stubbed your toe on. Parents may unconsciously think, "Why have you hurt me?" or, "Why did you stick me with this huge medical bill?" These reactions are futile. Such questions cannot be answered. The baby has no control over his situation. Even if he had, he would have chosen death rather than the heroic measures you or the doctor may have envisioned.

Often, it is not unusual to find relief following the death of a premature infant. Even though as a parent you may have kept your hopes up, in the back of your mind you anticipated death. The emotional stress, the worries, and the pressures that you were under have now been relaxed as a result of the death. The feeling is natural, and you should not trouble yourself accepting a sense of gladness along with sorrow. Some parents, however, are uncomfortable when they feel relieved that death may have been a solution to the seemingly insoluable problem of a preemie who may have been a "million dollar baby" who would have suffered serious, difficult-to-correct defects, or one that would have had to be institutionalized the rest of its life. It is hard for some parents to see anything good in death, especially the death of a child. As a result, they feel guilty when they have a perfect right to be grateful for the release that death can bring.

A parent's grief can take many forms, but no matter what form it takes, it is a personal thing. Although thousands have felt similar pain, they have not felt yours. You may find help in dealing with your grief—a preemie support group, your family, your church, even poetry. But the burden eventually returns for you to deal with personally. Perhaps the passage of time may be the most important factor in resolving your grief. But time only heals, it does not erase.

60. How should I tell my other children about my preemie's death?

If you have involved your other children with your situation all along, you shouldn't have too much of a problem. Certainly you shouldn't shield them. Death is sad, but sadness is an integral part of our lives.

Simply explain, in terms the child can understand, that the baby was just too small, too young, and not fully developed. Don't be afraid to cause tears; they are a safety valve. The expression of grief through tears and crying is normal and helpful. The worst possible thing is for the child to repress them. The child who keeps a firm lid on his grief may later have an explosive release that can be dangerous.

Although parents should not deny the child the opportunity to cry, neither should they urge siblings to display unfelt feelings. Remember, death is not as real to children as to adults, and the death of a preemie sibling seems even more distant because your other children will not have had as much contact with him as you have.

61. My premature baby died after a week in the intensive care nursery. I have a large bill, and no baby to show for it. Will I at least be able to deduct the medical expenses and claim my child that died as a dependent for that year?

Yes, you will be able to deduct the medical expenses (see next question), and yes, you will also be able to claim your child as a dependent, despite the fact that it lived for only a week. If it had lived for only a minute, you would still be able to claim the child as a dependent.

The Internal Revenue Service, in publication 501 (revised Nov., 1979), states:

> If your child was born alive during the year, and the dependency tests are met, you may take the full $1000 exemption.

This is true even if the child lived only for a moment. A child is considered to have lived if the state or local law treats the child as having been born alive. There must be proof to a live birth evidenced by an official document, such as a birth certificate. You may not claim an exemption for a stillborn child.

The key is having the necessary official document. Make certain that you have a birth certificate, even if the baby died only a few moments after birth. Such a consideration will not alleviate the grief you may feel, but it will ease the financial pain for that year.

62. Are there any other tax breaks parents of preemies should be aware of?

Because intensive nursery care is so expensive, the parents of a preemie may find themselves financially strapped for some time after the birth of their child, and every penny saved helps. There are indeed certain matters parents should be aware of for tax purposes.

First, you can only take the medical expenses of your premature child if you itemize your deductions. If you don't have medical insurance, or if there is a sizeable portion of the bill your insurance did not pay, the medical expenses themselves may be enough to warrant not using the short form. You should remember that the expenses incurred by the birth of your premature child must be claimed under "Schedule A" under the medical part of the tax form.

As for what is tax deductible, there is the obvious: hospital bills, doctors' bills, drugs, and medicines. But don't forget the less obvious. Mileage to and from the ICN or hospital is deductible at nine cents a mile, but this may change. Consult a current tax guide or the information booklet furnished by the IRS. Long distance phone calls to check on your child's condition, or to call the doctor or hospital, are deductible. If you have a doctor's suggestion (get it in writing) that your presence at the ICN will benefit either you or your baby, motel expenses, but not meals, will be deductible.

And don't forget special supplies. Perhaps the doctor suggests a humidifier, or you rented an electric breast pump—anything that is an unusual expense for most babies or is recommended by your doctor qualifies.

One final reminder—save all your cancelled checks and receipts in case you are audited, and you likely will be. Because your medical expenses will probably be unusually high, IRS computers will target your return for an audit. Many of my preemie parents endure audits. Falecia's parents did, but because of their records, they faced no problems. It may help to keep a kind of log or diary in which you note and record expenses and mileage.

chapter five

COMING HOME

A PARENT SPEAKS

We didn't know whether we would be bringing home a boy or a girl, we didn't know when we would be bringing our baby home, but we had resigned ourselves to accepting the baby for whatever she was or whatever she would become. What else could one do? The only other things we could do were to wait and worry. And while we waited and worried, we watched Falecia grow. We took pride in the fact that she was eating well, growing, and gaining weight. She still didn't yet weigh three pounds, but in comparison to what she had been, she seemed large to us. And yet there was always something that happened to put things in perspective.

Faye's sister had bought Falecia a baby ring with a tiny diamond, but it was far too large. She wouldn't be able to wear it until she was at least three or four. I put it in her hand, and sticking three of her fingers through it, she grasped it tightly.

"She knows diamonds are a girl's best friend," cracked the nurse, watching. We all laughed. "It would be impossible to find a ring small enough to fit her," she said.

"You may be right," I answered. "But you could make one."

Later, I took a piece of spare plastic hospital tubing and measured her ring finger. I could cut one out of a dime, but since dimes are no longer made of silver anyway, I decided to be chintzy and use a penny.

That night at home, with the plastic tube for a guide, I took a penny and started to bore a hole in it for her finger. I would have to grind a lot of that penny away for a ring that small. Then an inspired thought struck me! The tube was just about the size of a .22 caliber cartridge.

I found a spent casing, and sure enough! The tube easily slipped inside it. All I would have to do would be to cut the ring off the brass .22 casing. A hack saw did that job in seconds, and then I took my whetstone and carefully ground off the sharp edges. Next, I took some fine steel wool and polished it until it shone like new money. The brass took a finish like it was solid gold.

The new ring was so small that it could easily be lost, so I slipped it over the hospital tube and doubled it back on itself, making a coil so that it wouldn't slip off.

By now, it was past 1 A.M., and Faye, who lay reading in bed, remarked that it was some daughter we had who could wrap her father around her little finger like she did. I laughed and kissed her goodnight.

We didn't make it back to the ICN until two days later. Falecia had gained a full two ounces. She was up to 2 lbs. 15 ozs, and the ring was too small for the finger I had made it for, but it just fit her little finger. It would have to be a pinkie ring. She wore it only for the few minutes we and the nurses played with her and watched her. I knew that the next time we saw her, it wouldn't even fit her little finger. She would have outgrown it forever.

I was glad, and I put the ring in a safe place, along with the tiny diamond her aunt had gotten her. I didn't mind at all spending that time making a product whose practical use was so short-lived.

The next time we came up, Falecia weighed 3 lbs. Faye had baked a rum pound cake in celebration, and we brought it up for her surrogate mothers to have for their coffee break. There was enough for all three shifts of them.

Some of the nurses conspired to have some especially small clothes a friend had made and ultra-small pink booties knitted by a friend of Faye's sister taken down and sent through the sterilizer so that we could take a picture of Falecia in full dress. Previously, all the pictures I had taken had been "nudies," or shots of Falecia with her general issue preemie hospital gown on. The head nurse said they shouldn't have the clothes sterilized because of the unnecessary expense, but they were "accidentally" sent down anyway.

That evening, they dressed her up, and I took the first picture in which she was totally unencumbered—no wires, no monitors, no oxygen mask. She was held away from her oxygen for those few seconds it took me to take the pictures. Faye and the whole bunch of them reminded me of little girls playing with dolls. There wasn't that much difference between the two, except that their doll was alive and the girls were a bit older.

Falecia's lungs were becoming stronger, and Dr. Griesemer had been gradually dropping her oxygen level—28 percent, 27 percent, 26 percent, until finally she was down to 22 percent, just 1 percent above room air content. She remained at that mixture for several days, and then one evening we came up and found that she was on room air. It was a marvelous feeling, especially since her heart rate drops had totally disappeared. It had been a week since she had had a single one. She was on her road to coming home, except there was the cloud of the genetic test in the background.

Finally word came. The blood cells had failed to grow. They would have to have another sample and try again. So it was back to Falecia for another blood sample and more weeks of waiting.

By now, the strange and wonderous things that govern growth had been set in motion. Falecia's genitals changed almost overnight, and in a few days, it was obvious that the fat pads of labia were developing. Still, the genetic test would confirm our hopes. She also began developing even larger cheeks, and some of the nurses nicknamed her "Chipmunk." As her jaw muscles became stronger, she developed the sucking instinct. The little pacifier made for her by the nurses from a preemie-size bottle nipple became more interesting to her, and she would suck on it longer. If I lay my finger on her cheek, she would turn to it and try to nurse on it.

It was now time to see if Faye could feed her, and if Falecia could feed herself. Until now, she had been a "welfare baby," who didn't do anything for her food. She didn't even have to swallow it, because the gavage tube had been inserted and the milk simply poured in. Faye had been expressing her milk with an electric pump, which we joking called her Surge or DeLaval after the popular brands of milkers for large dairy herds. Faye had been freezing her milk, and we regularly made "milk runs" to the ICN at Cox for Falecia. Because Falecia required so little milk, and because Faye produced so much, the hospital's freezer and our home freezer were soon filled, and Faye had to start dumping it. We tried feeding some of it to our cat, Thomas Le Chat, but it gave him diarrhea. So gallons of what we believed had literally saved Falecia's life wound up in the city sewer.

At first, Falecia tired rapidly when feeding at the breast, but she tried valiantly. We would weigh her before and after feeding, to see how much she had taken, and what she couldn't take from the breast because she had exhausted herself, the nurses fed her by gavage tube. Gradually, as she gained strength and weight, she took more.

I had jokingly told Dr. Greisemer that we had to have Falecia out of the hospital and home by July 5, the day our insurance ran out. But that day had come and gone. We didn't expect to have her home until at least her due date, August 17, and perhaps even later. Five pounds was the magic number. The ICN staff and most pediatricians like babies to weigh at least that much. Janet, a friend who had gone to Europe for a summer vacation and planned to be back early in August, had said that she would give us a shower just before Falecia was released.

But Janet didn't get to plan the shower. She didn't even get to attend it. Dr. Griesemer and Falecia threw her plans, and ours, off schedule. She was doing so well that it would be some time in mid- or late July that Falecia would come home, and it would be before she weighed 5 lbs. We panicked. Faye had doubts about whether she could care for Falecia. Although she seemed large to us—in comparison to what she had been months earlier—she was still very small. And I learned that mothering is not just pure instinct. The nurses, who seemed to be so efficient and such good mothers, often had to release their charges to women, the true mothers, who actually caused me to feel sorry for the baby. A woman may be a biological parent, but that doesn't make her a good mother.

My mother called and told Faye how terrified she had been giving my brother Bob his first bath forty-six years ago. She said her heart had just thumped. I never expected such a remark from *my* mother, the old pro who raised six boys and mothered numerous neighbor children and grandchildren.

Faye began spending more time at the ICN, giving Falecia her bath, caring for her, and performing the usual and necessary duties of a mother. I told the nurses that they ought to give us at least a 50 percent reduction in the bill for those days because she was doing so much of their job! They said their tutoring fee would just equal my suggested 50 percent reduction, and so we were even. We began putting together the necessary things in anticipation of Falecia's arrival. I soon learned how expensive those items were, and I soon learned that if the nation's recycling program could duplicate the recycling system among our town's mothers, the drain on our natural resources would be cut to a minimum. The French professor provided a bed, changing table, buggy, and potty chair/trainer. My ex-college roommate promised a walker his daughter had outgrown. Another friend promised a tricycle his daughter had discarded. My sister-in-law provided a cradle my brother had built for her first child.

Plans for a shower were shouldered by Patty, who had become Falecia's godmother, Suzanne, Pat, and Lilly. Janet, who was in Italy, would be left out. Besides, we learned from a postcard from Rome, we would have to begin planning a shower for her later in the year! The shower, held in the faculty lounge and an adjoining room on campus, provided a study in the basic difference in the psychology of men and women. I was amazed how students and future mothers, mothers present, and mothers past provided gifts, both practical and impractical, jokes, and helpful hints. The whole affair seemed to be a kind of feminine ritual that launched the showeree officially into motherhood and reaffirmed their own role in the drama of the life process.

There were many frilly dresses, most of which were far too large, but Falecia would grow into them. There were gifts from casual acquaintances who had not been invited, but had given them to our friends to bring to the shower. There was a gift from a woman who had heard about Falecia in the laundromat from the wife of a colleague. And there was an original drawing of some kewpies by Rose O'Neill, the inventor of the kewpie doll, who had lived in the area years ago, from Faye's former supervising art teacher. There were hand-quilted baby blankets, afghans, and crocheted dresses, and diapers, dresses, and more diapers. If it weren't for baby showers and recycling, our society wouldn't be able to afford babies.

I showed them a series of slides I had taken that showed Falecia's progress from the ventilator, the CPAP, the oxyhood, the isolette, to a final picture of a little girl with dark hair, nursing and waiting to come home. Not one seemed bored by the home movies.

Although we looked forward to Falecia's homecoming, there were still several problems. For Faye, there was the concern about the pre-malignancy that had existed before her pregnancy. Enough time had passed so that she could have a D&C and have the uterine tissue tested. The weekend after the shower, she went into the hospital to have that done. Falecia had a problem with her eyes. They were constantly being checked, and her eye doctor was disturbed by the growth and proliferation of blood vessels in her eyes. In addition, she had a detached retina. One corner was loose and floating around in the fluid of the eyeball. There was the possibility that it would heal. If not, surgery would have to be performed at some future date, and a laser beam would be used to attach the retina by means of scar tissue. So we waited more—for Falecia's eyes to improve, for the results of the genetic test, and for the lab report on Faye's precancerous condition.

Faye stayed with my niece and her husband in Springfield and went to the hospital for Falecia's feedings. I stayed at home and taught my classes and make lots of phone calls to Springfield. My students would usually start my classes with the question, "When is your daughter coming home?" And the same question was asked each noon in the faculty lounge at the bridge table. My answer was always, "Soon."

A DOCTOR SPEAKS

63. When will I get to take my baby home?

The answer to that question depends on the baby's doctor and the baby. When the treatment for any illness, or prematurity, is completed, when the weight nears five pounds, when the baby can maintain its body temperature, is eating well and gaining weight, and when you as a parent have shown the necessary skill and competence in feeding and caring, the baby is ready to graduate from the world of the ICN to the greater world.

64. Will I have to turn up the heat, get a humidifier, or do anything special when my preemie comes home?

Unless your child had special, serious problems, you won't have to do anything different for your premature child than for a full-term baby. Temperature control for the baby remains a concern at home, just as it was in the hospital. Before the baby is discharged, a lot of effort goes into determining that the baby can maintain a temperature of 98°–99° without the help of an incubator. The temperature of your house is best regulated for the baby simply by maintaining the thermostat in the range you find most comfortable for yourself. The addition of a light blanket for the baby will help make minor fluctuations in room temperature tolerable for the baby. Keep the baby out of windy, draft-prone areas.

If you live in a climate that makes your home dry in the winter, it is often a good idea to buy a humidifier. It will be better for you and your baby. However, there is really no need to have a humidifier installed in your heating system. A simple, inexpensive room humidifier for the baby's room will be more than adequate.

65. Should I take my preemie outside?

The answer depends on what problems your child had and what time of the year your baby arrives home. If no breathing problems persist, and it isn't the middle of winter, the baby will tolerate short trips outside with an appropriate covering. If it is cold and your child did have breathing problems during his or her ICN stay, it would be better to stay inside.

Certainly as the weather warms, you should take your child outside. Sunlight is good for children, and the stimulation an outside environment provides will encourage your child's mental development.

66. When will I be able to take my premature baby out in public?

Specific situations depend on your baby, your physician's advice, and you. In general, you would be wise to keep the premature infant somewhat cloistered and away from other small children until the 9–10 lbs. range is reached. Children in the younger age range often can be well one hour and sick the next, and it would be easy for them to carry a rather serious childhood disease and be totally unaware that they are sick or a carrier. By establishing a "No Children" rule, you can prevent lots of unnecessary exposure.

Likewise, you might want to limit adult company. Your friends and neighbors will be excited and interested when you bring your premature baby home, probably more so than if he or she had been born full-term. People are attracted to small things—baby animals, toy trains, and tiny babies. They may mean well, but frequent visitors and frequent handling of the baby can tire both of you. Remember, your first duty is to yourselves and your child. Allow only visitors and social duties that you can handle. Remember that friends and visitors will want what is best for you and the baby. A simple word of explanation to them will make matters easier for you.

67. Are there any dangers I should be aware of when I take my premature baby home?

Yes, as parents, you should be aware of being overly concerned about your child. Your doctor and the ICN would not release the baby if the risks were too great. You should take all normal, sensible precautions with your child, but you should try not to develop what is called the *Vulnerable Child Syndrome*.

The Vulnerable Child Syndrome is a disturbed interaction pattern of behavior which reflects concern by the parents for an earlier life-threatening illness of the child. The responses of parents who suffer from this syndrome are overprotectiveness, fears that the child might stop breathing or is afflicted with a weak heart, concern about the child's weight gain, and a reluctance to leave the child with a baby sitter.

If you find that you are reacting to your child in such a way that would seem unusual if the baby had not been premature, you would do well to examine your behavior. Treat the premature baby as you would any other baby. It will help both of you.

68. Now that my premature baby is home, I am afraid to handle her. Her smallness scares me.

Of course her smallness scares you. What also scares you is a fear that you won't handle her right, coupled with the idea that babies, especially premature babies, are frail and delicate. Babies are not all that frail, and a premature baby, by the time that it gets to go home, is, for all practical purposes, a newborn. If the baby was so delicate that handling it would be harmful, the hospital would not have discharged the baby. Frequent visits to the nursery and participating as much as possible in your infant's care serves as good training.

As for handling the premature baby, the normal precautions should be followed. Supporting the head of a premature infant is especially important because the neck muscles develop slowly. The soft spot on the top of the skull (called the anterior fontanel), is actually protected by a tough membrane. Parents often worry needlessly about this soft spot on the head, which closes as the bones in the skull grow and mature.

69. I didn't send birth announcements while my premature child was in the ICN. Now, three months later, she is home and I'm not sure what to do. Should I send announcements now?

Pediatricians aren't usually asked questions about etiquette, but your question is certainly legitimate. Elizabeth L. Post, probably America's best-known etiquette authority , suggests you wait until the baby is out of danger before sending birth announcements. Her advice is to use regular announcements, filling in the birth date and other information, adding a line to say that your baby has just arrived home from the hospital. Another of her suggestions is for you to announce the baby's "homecoming."

Her advice is sound. First, you will be worried about your baby while it is in the hospital, and you probably won't even have time to send announcements. Second, if there is a real concern that your preemie may not survive, it is best to delay any announcements because your friends may not know how to react to an announcement that indicates a definite low-weight birth. You thus avoid putting them in an awkward position.

A birth announcement is a sharing of your joy. Delaying the announcement until the baby comes home solves many problems and makes the announcement of your little miracle even more joyous.

70. How can I expect my other children to react when I bring my preemie home?

This question merits considerable attention because siblings often feel neglected as the attention of parents is quite naturally focused on the premature family arrival. Older children often react in a negative, hostile manner when a younger brother or sister is born, and these natural feelings can be intensified by a preemie.

First, let's examine reactions of siblings from the very beginning—when the premature birth disrupts family life. Younger brothers and sisters may find that their parents' attention and concerns for the new arrival puts them, in a sense, on the back burner. Parents may be away at the hospital much of the time, and the children are left in the care of relatives or a sitter. Parents have less time to play with siblings, and less time to read to them. Siblings find that all talk and attention is directed to the preemie.

This neglect can result in two possible reactions. The siblings may regress and act more childish in order to get attention. A toilet-trained child may all of a sudden become untrained. He may cry more frequently, be cranky, and demand attention, often in exasperating ways, such as throwing toys or spilling his milk. Such behavior is hostile reaction expressing itself in a covert manner. But sometimes this hostility expresses itself in a more open manner: The child may actively say things about his premature sibling to show his feelings, or he may express his actions physically—by hitting, pinching, or in other ways mistreating his new brother or sister.

Sometimes the child reacts to the premature birth in an unusual way: He feels guilty and responsible for the premature birth and all the grief and problems it may have caused his parents. He may develop feelings of inferiority and guilt, he may regress, or he may have nightmares. If such a guilt reaction happens, it may express itself in a variety of ways, but the child will be thoroughly unhappy in any event.

Parents should be especially aware from the beginning about possible sibling problems and take action to prevent them. First, explain to the children exactly what happened and what caused it. You may not know for certain yourself, and if you do, a detailed explanation isn't necessary. What is necessary is that the child is made aware that the situation isn't his fault.

Second, don't neglect your other children. It may be difficult, but make room for them in your hectic life while your preemie is in the hospital. Find time to play with them, to read to them, and to take them out for activities. It may be difficult, but the time will be well-spent, not only for them, but for you. Your other children may take your mind off your problems.

Lastly, involve your children in the situation. Explain to them not only what happened, but what is going on. The unknown and the secret generate fear and distrust. Explanations and involvement can dissipate sibling fears. If possible, take your children into the ICN to see the new arrival. If ICN policy does not permit such an activity, allow your children to view their new brother or sister through the window. Show them pictures you have taken. Keep them posted about progress. Have them make or buy a toy for the child. Have the ICN sterilize their gift, and place it in the incubator with the preemie sibling. Let your children know the child got the gift by letting them see it in the incubator or by taking a picture of it in the incubator. Explain to them that their interest and concern will help their new brother or sister come home earlier.

Such involvement will prevent problems and will make the

homecoming easier for all involved, you, your preemie child, and just as importantly, your other children.

71. When will my premature baby get all his immunizations and shots?

The battery of immunizations and shots that have become common to protect babies from the diseases that used to ravage children will not begin until your baby is able to stand the stress of them. Generally, that will be after he is home and when he weighs at least six pounds. Your pediatrician will suggest a date for your baby's immunizations when the baby is released from the ICN. In general, premature infants receive the same number and kind of immunizations given to full-term infants.

72. My premature child seems to cry much more than my other two children. Are there any effective methods for calming and soothing him?

In a recent study, Dr. Sarah Friedman and her research colleagues at the National Institute of Mental Health found that pre-term babies, at the time they would have been born if carried to full term, are more irritable and less easy to soothe than full-term newborns. As time goes by, some parents may find their pre-term babies become easier to soothe.

All parents, whether their babies be pre- or full-term, are interested in baby-calming techniques. One of the simplest and most effective calming techniques is swaddling, which means wrapping a baby securely from shoulders to feet with a small blanket or sheet, much in the way Indian mothers wrap their papooses. While parents may feel uncomfortable about restricting the movement of their infants' arms and legs in this way, Drs. Earle L. Lipton, Alfred Sternschneider, and Julius B. Richmond found that swaddling for limited periods seems to soothe babies. No one is sure why swaddling is such an effective calmer. Possibly it gives a baby a sense of security to be tightly wrapped, or maybe it is the sensory stimulation of the blanket or sheet on the baby's skin. Researchers have found that various other types of sensory stimulation—certain sounds and movements, for instance—seem to calm babies. Although parents may not have realized they were stimulating their baby's senses by holding, rocking, singing, and talking to them, they have long used these techniques to soothe their infants.

Another relatively simple way of calming babies has been discovered by parents who use a modern version of the papoose carrier. Today's mothers and fathers can be seen going about their activities with an apparently contented baby snuggled in a carrier strapped to the parent's back or chest. Mothers are reporting that the carriers are not only convenient toters but seem to be effective calmers. Apparently the carriers offer a baby a combination of comforts, closeness to the parent, the sensory stimulation of swaddling, and physical motion.

73. My premature baby cries a lot and doubles up his legs. He seems to have the colic. Do premature babies get colic?

Many physicians feel that colic results from air being trapped in the infant's intestine, causing cramping and discomfort. Infants who eat quickly, eat large volumes, or swallow air directly or mixed with food, seem to be more prone to get colic. Premature infants who begin growing very quickly also attempt to catch up on their feedings, even when the muscles associated with swallowing are not fully developed and are more prone to cause increased amounts of air to be swallowed with the feedings. Consequently, colic seems to be an added problem with premature infants, even though many doctors doubt the condition truly exists.

You may suspect your baby has colic if he is dry, full, burped, and warm, but still crying. Some signs of colic are: severe crying, reddening of the face, pulling of the legs up to the abdomen, and the clenching of fists. Babies who have colic are obviously uncomfortable. Attacks seem to start suddenly, can last many hours, and stop just as suddenly. They may last intermittently for days, with the baby resting only after he has literally worn himself out. In some babies, attacks seem to occur about the same time every day or night.

What can you do? Be patient. You will find burping your baby after every feeding, keeping the head slightly elevated after feeding, and letting the baby lie on his or her stomach with the legs tucked underneath to be helpful. Gentle massage of the baby's back, added warmth, and lots of cuddling are also a help. None of these things may cure the colic, but they will make your baby (and you) feel a lot better. As the infant matures and the growth rate slows, the problems with colic fade.

Recently many medications previously used for colic have been scrutinized more closely, especially with regard to their use in premature infants. Neonatologists strongly recommend not using any medication for colic in a premature infant—particularly brandy and other liquors—without consulting with your physician.

74. My premature baby is often sick and cries a lot, and I am ashamed to say that I actually find myself wanting to deliberately hurt her. Sometimes I even do. What can I do?

Being aware of the problem and actively seeking help are the only things you can do. As a rational human being who is really concerned about the welfare of your child, but who expresses emotions in ways that may actually harm the baby, you will want to be aware of certain information so that you can make the best decisions for your child.

Studies show that a fairly high proportion of abused children were born prematurely. Studies also indicate that parents who abuse their children often were the victims of abuse when they were children. In turn, they become abusing adults, particularly when they are under stress. Abusing parents often do not have the close ties to family, friends, and community that might provide them help when they have problems. Because of the stresses involved in having and caring for a pre-term baby, you may wish to seek help. Hospital-based social workers are often available to help parents cope with stress and to arrange other needed services, such as financial aid or home visits from a public health nurse.

Another source of information and assistance is a mutual help group with which parents of pre-term babies meet regularly to share experiences and knowledge. Studies indicate that parents participating in such a group, which is usually organized and assisted by a staff nurse, are providing better care and appear more at ease with their babies than parents who do not participate. When such groups are not organized by hospital staff, parents may want to take the initiative and form a mutual help group.

Calling on willing family members and friends for needed relief is also good for a new parent. If money is not a problem, the services of a capable baby sitter may help tremendously. The important issue is that you acknowledge your need for help and ask for it freely, without guilt, before reaching the end of your rope.

75. What should I do about a baby sitter?

First, get a baby sitter. It is important that you have a break from the cares and problems of the pre-term infant. Being a parent is probably the most important job there is, and you'll do a better job if you get to take a coffee break periodically.

Baby-sitting is a worry. As the parents of a premature baby, you have learned so much about prematurity that you may find it hard to leave your baby for even a short time with someone else. Some parents hire a nurse as a baby sitter. Others feel comfortable with another member of the family. And some parents of premature babies baby-sit for each other.

It will be difficult, but you must take the plunge. As the baby gets older, you will find that your feelings of anxiety will be lessened, and pretty soon you will think nothing of leaving your former preemie with the teen-age sitter from up the street.

76. What problems will I have relating to my premature child?

The parents of a premature child have tremendous adjustments to make. During the pregnancy, there is a psychological preparation that normally involves the wish for an impossibility—a perfect child. There is also the corresponding dread of a damaged one. Adjusting to the discrepancy between the perfect child conceived only in the mind and the premature child that actually exists is one of the tasks of the parents, if a healthy parent-child relationship is to be developed.

After the birth of a premature child, the parents must prepare themselves for the fact that the child may die. They must also accept the fact that they have not produced a normal, full-term infant, and certainly not the perfect baby they dreamed of. Next, the parents must begin interacting with the infant that has been born and face the reality of their situation. And finally, they must become aware of the infant's special needs so that they can act with constructiveness and sensitivity in fulfilling those needs.

77. What kinds of parents best manage to accept a premature child?

Parents who seem to manage well in the intensive care nursery are those who have a stable marriage, are in their late twenties or early thirties, have support from family, friends, or community and strong religious beliefs, and who are good at actively seeking information from the ICN staff and their child's pediatrician. The parents who best manage to accept their un-perfect child are verbal, intelligent, and have an understanding of their child's medical problems.

You may not have all the characteristics of the ideal parents of a preemie, but you will have some of them, and this book certainly should provide information about your situation and your child's situation. You can help yourself and your child by actively seeking information from the ICN staff. They will be glad to help you.

chapter six

FUTURE CONCERNS

A PARENT SPEAKS

Falecia's homecoming approached rapidly. Both Faye and I were busy, but in the back of our minds lurked worries about the problem with Falecia's eyes and the genetic test. Even further back in our minds, but rapidly coming to the front, were questions about the future, about Falecia's mental and social development in the years to come. Would she have trouble learning to talk? Would Falecia have learning disabilities or be a slow learner? Would she ever catch up in her physical development? There were so many questions for the future. However, the problems of the present pushed aside our worries and questions for the time being. Faye spent all the time she could at the hospital with Falecia, spending more time there than at her niece's home where she was staying.

I stayed busy at home. The last week of my temporary bachelorhood was filled with grading papers, reading for my classes, and plotting a southern, gothic novel—a wild and probably fruitless scheme to help pay Falecia's hospital bills. Faye would call every evening to report on Falecia's and her own progress as she learned to care for the daughter that would soon be her own. One evening she reported that the genetic test had come back perfect and normal in every way. Falecia's eyes were better because the blood vessels looked more normal, but the detached retina of the left eye was no better. However, it also was no worse.

And the results of Faye's uterine tissue test had also come back. No abnormality or malignancy was found in any of the tissues. What an evening! Why the change in the prepregnancy test and the postpregnancy test? Faye had always felt that Falecia had cured her condition. Perhaps it was so. On the other hand, pre-cancerous and cancerous cells change or die for no apparent reason. Who knows what caused the change?

And so on a Friday, two days before Falecia would be three months old and twenty-one days before her scheduled birth, she got to come home. She was now a whopping four pounds, five ounces. We had agreed to let the Cox Medical Center use Falecia, their smallest survivor, to promote their planned new intensive care nursery. News of her scheduled release was featured on all the Springfield radio stations, and she promoted a new and better facility than the one that had saved her life so that smaller and younger babies with far more serious problems could be saved. She had begun paying her debt to the hospital, her nurses, and society. The handbook for parents of preemies that she inspired was coming along nicely. Perhaps she would be able to help parents as well as their children. Falecia was the subject of a long article in the Springfield paper and in her own local paper. It was amazing that such a little girl could be such big news, but people hunger for "dessert news," or stories that make them feel good or that have a happy ending.

I released my last class that Friday a bit early, and my friend John once again loaned me his station wagon for the trip home. His wife, Suzanne, came along to chauffeur, and Patty came along for the ride, and to provide any needed assistance. It was rather appropriate that the Pontiac station wagon that had taken Falecia to the hospital to be born almost three months earlier should be bringing her home. And appropriate also was the fact that this time she was coming home in the front seat.

At the hospital, the newspaper photographer was finishing the last of his pictures and talking to Faye. Kathy, one of the nurses, had made Falecia a special homecoming dress, and her assigned nurse of the day, Daylene, put it on her for Falecia's official nursery release photograph. All of her odds and ends were put on a hospital cart, along with the usual freebies from baby products manufacturers. Faye had to read the ID number on Falecia's bracelet so Daylene could check her hospital birth record, to see if they matched. "What if they don't match?" I asked. "Do we still get to take her home?"

"No, we just give you one of the other babies who didn't match up. It all comes out even in the end," she joked.

In the elevator, Daylene gave Falecia a goodbye kiss.

"Isn't that unprofessional and against hospital policy?" I joked.

"This is the first time in almost three months that I've succumbed," she said. "I don't think that is too bad."

I thought of all Falecia's other mothers at the ICN. I wondered if they would miss the senior citizen of the ICN, or if they soon become just as attached to her replacements? I hoped so. I also wondered if Nurse Debbie, who had no children of her own and who had taken a special interest in Falecia, had deliberately called in sick that day so that she would not have to see Falecia leave.

Daylene carried Falecia down the hall. It was official hospital policy. Babies are not given to the mother until she is in the car. As we walked down the corridor, I thought of a colleague in my department at the college, whose father had died in this same hospital just the night before. As I pushed Falecia's cart, I glanced into one of the rooms. An old woman, wrinkled and tired, who must have been at least ninety, and who had probably come to the hospital to die, saw Daylene carrying Falecia and smiled. The smile must have been to herself, as there was no one in the room with her. Perhaps Falecia had made her day just a bit more pleasant. The situation was ironic: The aged woman, coming to the hospital "to go home," and Falecia, young enough not to have been born yet, leaving the hospital to go home. The cycles of the centuries and the success of the human species were contained in that single moment in that single smile.

Back home, the neighborhood children, who were as interested in Falecia as were their parents, had tied pink streamers on the trees that lined our street. A sign in one yard offered its congratulations, and our mailbox was decorated with a large pink bow. Pink balloons and streamers festooned the front porch, and a large sign in the yard announced to the world, "Falecia Lives Here!" Covering the garage door, another touted its message: "Welcome Home, Falecia!" I took Faye's picture as she held Falecia in front of it.

Later, flocks of neighborhood parents and children came down to take a look at her through the picture window, a precaution suggested by Dr. Griesemer. He didn't want to expose her to the germs of the entire world until she weighed about eight pounds. As they smiled, oohing and ahing, through the window, I thought of all the changes I had seen in Falecia during the last three months, of the long hours, the lost sleep, and the neglected work. I thought of all the work, effort, technology, knowledge, and prayers that made Falecia's homecoming possible. I remembered the note we had found attached to her crib by her nurses at the hospital: "Dear Mom and Dad: Guess what!? My chart weighs 5 lbs. 6 oz., and that's not even all of it. I am trying to catch up to my chart!" I wondered how long it would take her to catch up. I thought of the computerized printout with every lab test, tube, and bottle accounted for. Faye's hospital stay had produced a printout three feet long. Falecia's would probably be three miles long! She hadn't cost as much as Dr. Griesemer had forecast, but if I were to add Faye's bills because of the pregnancy, the pediatrician's bills, the specialists' bills, and the hospital bill, Falecia's per ounce cost, calculated on her birth weight of one pound and eight ounces, was $2833.33 per ounce. And she was worth every penny of it.

Thinking back over it all, the problems of the past seemed almost a dream, and the concerns for the future once again came to mind. It had been a very long road to this moment, but it was only a beginning.

A DOCTOR SPEAKS

78. Now that my premature child's survival is assured, I have started worrying about the baby's development. Do I have a cause for worry?

You, the grandparents, and your friends will marvel and express wonder at your child's smallness. Small babies are cute babies, and premature children attract lots of attention. But after the initial attention your baby and you receive, there comes a point when you will begin to wonder and worry about your child's development. This concern is natural, but it is often a concern that doesn't strike the parents for days, weeks, or even months (as in the case of Falecia's parents) after the baby is born.

You may expect your child to look small in comparison to other children her age for quite some time, even years. In fact, some teachers in kindergarten and first grade can spot a preemie child simply because the child may be so much smaller and more delicate looking than her peers. However, a preemie's physical growth tends to overtake full-term babies by the second or third year. As for mental development, the greater the immaturity and the lower the birth weight, the greater the likelihood of intellectual and nervous disorders. Follow-up studies of preemie survivors indicate a high incidence of handicaps among the smaller ones. In addition, behavior and personality problems appear to be more common in children born prematurely.

Even with today's medical technology, some pre-term infants will have problems in the future. The percentage of children with severe problems, such as blindness, cerebral palsy, or serious mental retardation, has been sharply reduced by modern intensive care medicine, just as survival rates have increased for those with very low birth weights and other severe complications. However, according to recent research findings, serious problems continue to be reported for about 4 percent to 8 percent of infants whose birth weight is less than 3 1/3 lbs.

Some pre-term infants, particularly those with respiratory diseases, may be vulnerable to respiratory problems like pneumonia later in life. Others, particularly those with the lowest birth weights or other severe neonatal problems, may be likely to develop milder disabilities such as hyperactivity, language lags, or learning disorders that may require special attention. In general, the most severe problems can be recognized soon after birth, but the milder problems are not obvious until early childhood.

To avoid unnecessary anxiety, parents should have their child checked regularly by a pediatrician or a local health clinic. If they are concerned about the early development of their infant, parents may want to get the help of a specialist who can evaluate his or her development on a regular basis.

79. My premature child is home now, but I'm afraid he won't be normal. How should I treat him?

First of all, be realistic and optimistic. Treat him as if he is normal so as not to cause further delays in development. Even if you know for certain your child is damaged in some manner, accept him for what he is, how he looks, or what he has. Do not dwell on something he doesn't have. If you can do that—and it may be a great task—you will be doing more for your child than if you were able to buy him anything he desired or anything you desired for him. If you can accept him and appreciate him for what he is, he will develop the confidence and strength he needs to face the problems he will encounter in the world. A child who is never quite accepted by a parent or parents always feels that he is not quite right. He will always lack the necessary self-confidence to make use of the talents, skills, and brains that he does have. A parent who does not accept the handicap his premature child has can only intensify and multiply that handicap as he grows up.

80. Will my premature child have difficulty getting health insurance? Will I have difficulty purchasing life insurance for my preemie?

Unless your child was born very prematurely or had serious medical problems and complications, you should have no difficulty purchasing life insurance on your child. Neither should your preemie have difficulty purchasing health insurance later in life. As for current health insurance, most policies automatically include coverage of the child when it is born, if that coverage is applied for within thirty days after the birth. To be on the safe side, check to see exactly what your policy says regarding health insurance coverage. Also, alert your agent or insurance company when the child is born. You may want to insure the child even before its birth. Most insurance companies have such a provision. However, that information doesn't do you any good now that your child is here and not insured.

If your child was born quite prematurely and/or had serious medical problems, the insurance company will probably want to do some investigative research before it issues a life insurance policy. Remember, even a $10,000 policy represents a substantial gamble by the company, and it does not want to have to pay off if it loses. You might keep in mind that when you buy life insurance, the company is gambling that you will live. It will want to check the odds. The insuring company will probably ask for an attending physician's form. This form asks certain routine questions to determine the risks— questions about heart and respiratory problems, for example. The company may also ask for X-rays and EKG results. A full medical exam may be requested. When you apply for the insurance, you automatically give the company the legal right to investigate your child's health. Such an investigation is paid for by the insurance company. It does not cost you anything, except perhaps increased administrative costs that will be spread, as increased premiums, among all customers. The important thing to remember is not to hide any problems. If you do and are later caught, you may have difficulty collecting.

For the most part, you don't have to worry. Most preemies do not have trouble buying insurance, although the premiums may be slightly higher for those who may have had serious medical problems and complications.

81. I know that my premature baby will have problems, but is there really anything I can do?

Studies of pre-term babies indicate that those who suffer severe medical complications tend to be more sluggish, less responsive, and more irritable than those who have had normal medical histories.

Also, researchers have conjectured that pre-term babies, who must remain hospitalized for relatively long periods of time, may be deprived of the benefits of mutual stimulation between parent and child. That is, pre-term babies and their parents have less opportunity to learn from and teach each other through social interactions. For example, when a baby cries or smiles, parents respond in specific ways. They may feed, hold, talk to, or smile at their babies. Babies learn from their parents' responses that they are loved, that they have some control over their world, and that specific behaviors elicit specific responses. Parents, in turn, learn about their babies' needs and personalities through observation and contact with them. Thus, through a process of mutual discovery, parents and babies learn to interact with each other.

If a baby has suffered severe medical complications and has had to remain in the hospital for weeks or months, the mutual learning process between parent and infant may be delayed or blunted. The lack of responsiveness and irritability of the baby may make him more difficult to care for. Nevertheless, many parents have found ways to overcome the difficulties. Researchers have found that an important factor in how well the pre-term infant, or any baby, for that matter, develops is the parents' attitudes and behaviors. Parents who persistently try to make eye contact with their babies, who talk to them during feedings, who hold them and rock them, and who, in general, interact more with their babies eventually are rewarded by their babies' responses and healthy development.

This is not to say that parents should exhaust or frustrate themselves trying to interact with their babies. They need to keep in mind that their baby may not be biologically ready to respond. On the other hand, some extra effort by parents to stimulate their babies may prove advantageous for their future development.

82. Now that my premature baby is home, are there any books or materials that will be of special help?

Unfortunately, there isn't much published material on preemies for parents. This book is designed to be of help from the time you have the premature child until you get the child home. You may have occasion to refer to it as your child develops. As for most baby development books, most preemie parents are wise to either toss them aside or read them with a grain of salt, keeping in mind that their child will not mirror the development of a full-term baby. Some preemie parents find such books distressing and worry themselves needlessly about their baby's slow development. If the book says the baby should be stacking blocks at age six months and their baby isn't, they may frustrate themselves and the baby by trying to teach him to stack blocks when he isn't interested or ready. I use the blocks as an example because a doctor friend of mine, a general practitioner, had premature twin boys. One evening he checked their progress against the Denver Developmental Test and found that they should be stacking blocks at that age. He spent an entire evening wearing out himself and the two boys, trying to show them how to stack blocks when all they were interested in was grasping them and biting them. Two months later, they were ready to stack blocks. That was seven years ago, and both are now doing well in school.

As for the general care of your baby, I would recommend the bible of baby care, Dr. Benjamin Spock's *Baby and Child Care.* It is a classic, and it is available in an inexpensive paperback edition by Pocket Books. You can find it in most book stores or drug stores.

83. I know that my premature child will have developmental problems. Besides your handbook, are there any other sources of information that I may find helpful along these lines?

Yes, there are. I would suggest you try your local library first. Libraries often have books about development or specific developmental problems. The more you learn about your child's problem, the better you will be able to help him. After your premature child is two to three years old, most of the information written in developmental books can be applied to him. Three books by the publisher of this handbook that can be helpful are:

A Child With a Problem: A Guide to the Psychological Disorders of Childhood, by Rainer Twiford (Region I Mental Health Center, MS). Describes in simple terms, the systems, causes, and prognosis of such disorders as autism, hyperactivity, and mental retardation. The author reveals scientific strategies for dealing with such behavior problems as bed-wetting, aggression, and delinquency. Included in this guide is up-to-date information on where and when to seek professional help, and what to expect on the first office visit.

Better Learning: Minor and Severe; From Five to Fifty, by Rosalie M. Young and Harriet H. Savage, Foreword by Mary G. Rockefeller. Explains how to reduce learning problems from preschool years to adulthood. Includes discussions on variations in learning, how children develop ideas, what kinds of problems surface in adolescence, and what maturity level and basic skills are needed for specific grades.

Special Children, Special Parents, by Albert T. Murphy. Offering support, insight, and guidance, this book provides concrete examples of the special emotions and unique personal relationships in the everyday lives of families with handicapped children.

In addition, you may write your local chapter of the Mental Health Association. Information about the Association can be obtained by writing to:

The Mental Health Association
1800 North Kent St.
Arlington, VA 22209

If you know what kind of problem *your* child has, there are a number of sources for information. By writing to the agencies and services for exceptional children listed below and asking for specific or general information, you should obtain either the information you desire or the source where you may obtain it.

Alexander Graham Bell Association for the Deaf, Inc.
Volta Bureau for the Deaf
3417 Volta Place, NW
Washington, DC 20007

American Academy of Pediatrics
1801 Hinman Ave.
Evanston, IL 60204

American Association on Mental Deficiency
5201 Connecticut Ave., NW
Washington, DC 20015

American Association of Psychiatric Clinics for Children
250 West 57th St.
New York, NY

American Bar Association Commission on the Mentally Disabled
1800 M St., NW
Washington, DC 20036

American Foundation for the Blind
15 W. 16th St.
New York, NY 10011

American Medical Association
535 N. Dearborn St.
Chicago, IL 60610

American Speech and Hearing Association
9030 Old Georgetown Road
Washington, DC 20014

Association for the Aid of Crippled Children
345 E. 46th St.
New York, NY 10017

Association for Children with Learning Disabilities
2200 Brownsville Road
Pittsburgh, PA 15210

Association for Education of the Visually Handicapped
1604 Spruce St.
Philadelphia, PA 19103

Association for the Help of Retarded Children
200 Park Ave., South
New York, NY

Association for the Visually Handicapped
1839 Frankfort Ave.
Louisville, KY 40206

Center on Human Policy
Division of Special Education and Rehabilitation
Syracuse University
Syracuse, NY 13210

Child Fund
275 Windsor St.
Hartford, CT 06120

Children's Defense Fund
1520 New Hampshire Ave., NW
Washington, DC 20036

Closer Look
National Information Center for the Handicapped
1201 Sixteenth St., NW
Washington, DC 20036

Clifford W. Beers Guidance Clinic
432 Temple St.
New Haven, CT 06510

Child Study Center
Yale University
333 Cedar St.
New Haven, CT 06520

Child Welfare League of America, Inc.
44 East 23rd St.
New York, NY 10010

Children's Bureau
United States Department of Health, Education and Welfare
Washington, DC

Council for Exceptional Children
1411 Jefferson Davis Highway
Arlington, VA 22202

Developmental Disabilities Office
Room 3070, 330 C St., SW
Washington, DC 20201

Epilepsy Foundation of America
1828 L St., NW
Washington, DC 20036

Family Service Association of America
401 M St., SW
Washington, DC 20460

Institute for the Study of Mental Retardation
and Related Disabilities
130 South First
University of Michigan
Ann Arbor, MI 48108

International Association for the Scientific Study
of Mental Deficiency
Ellen Horn, AAMD
5201 Connecticut Ave., NW
Washington, DC 20015

International League of Societies for the Mentally Handicapped
Rue Forestiere 12
Brussels, Belgium

Joseph P. Kennedy, Jr. Foundation
1701 K St., NW
Washington, DC 20006

League for Emotionally Disturbed Children
171 Madison Ave.
New York, NY

Muscular Dystrophy Associations of America
1790 Broadway
New York, NY 10019

National Aid to the Visually Handicapped
3201 Balboa St.
San Francisco, CA 94121

National Association of Coordinators of State Programs
for the Mentally Retarded
2001 Jefferson Davis Highway
Arlington, VA 22202

National Association of Hearing and Speech Agencies
919 18th St., NW
Washington, DC 20006

National Association for Creative Children and Adults
8080 Springfield Drive
Cincinnati, OH 45236

National Association for Retarded Citizens
2709 Avenue E East
Arlington, TX 76010

National Children's Rehabilitation Center
P.O. Box 1260
Leesburg, VA

National Association for the Visually Handicapped
3201 Balboa St.
San Francisco, CA 94121

National Association of the Deaf
814 Thayer Ave.
Silver Spring, MD 20910

National Cystic Fibrosis Foundation
3379 Peachtree Road NE
Atlanta, GA 30326

National Easter Seal Society for Crippled Children and Adults
2023 W. Ogden Ave.
Chicago, IL 60601

National Federation of the Blind
218 Randolph Hotel
Des Moines, IA 50309

National Paraplegia Foundation
333 N. Michigan Ave.
Chicago, IL 60601

National Society for Autistic Children
621 Central Ave.
Albany, NY 12206

National Society for Prevention of Blindness, Inc.
78 Madison Ave.
New York, NY 10016

Orton Society, Inc.
8415 Bellona Lane
Baltimore, MD 21264

President's Commission on Mental Retardation/OHD
7th & D St., SW
Washington, DC 20201

Society for Protection of the Unborn Through Nutrition (SPUN)
17 N. Wabash, Suite 603
Chicago, IL 60602

United Cerebral Palsy Association
66 E 34th St.
New York, NY 10016

84. What is the long view for my premature child? What can I expect?

Doctors cannot yet accurately predict the future of a pre-term, low-weight, or seriously ill newborn. Medical advances are too recent to gauge their long-term impact on children who have had the advantage of treatment in intensive care nurseries. But recent findings give parents reason to be optimistic. The majority of children studied, who now range in age from two to nine years of age, are free of serious problems. Because doctors cannot predict accurately a particular baby's future, parents may suffer needless worry when they ask a question like, "Will my child be retarded?" The physician's honest answer of, "Possibly" or, "I don't know yet" may be heard by stressed parents as a "yes" instead of a "maybe." It may or may not help parents who are worried about the future of their own baby to know that 75 percent of premature babies develop normally.

Doctors have found it important to repeat needed information on a number of occasions. Information that cannot be understood at first may be heard and understood at some later date when the parents are under less strain. Likewise, parents may have to ask the same questions more than once to get needed information. Also, parents who are told that their pre-term babies will catch up may become worried when they observe that their babies are developmentally slower than other babies born around the same time. They may not realize that their babies are really younger than full-term babies who were born on the same day. A pre-term baby's development should be considered on the basis of conceptual age rather than birth date. A baby that is born two months before term is always two months younger than the full-term baby born on the same day, and allowances should be made for this difference. Furthermore, all children—pre-term and full-term—develop at their own rates. The most important thing to look for in children is steady developmental progress, rather than specific age-related accomplishments.

On the average, children who were born before term are more apt to remain physically smaller than their full-term peers. Nevertheless, inherited genes and proper nutrition become the most important determinants of the child's physical size. Size has little to do with a child's capabilities, but adults tend to baby small children and expect too much from those who are large for their age. Children have a tendency to live up to adults' expectations and do best when they are expected to behave according to their capabilities rather than their size.

85. Will my premature child, mentally and physically, be behind children who were born full-term?

As a parent of a premature child, you must face certain facts. With all the marvels of medical science and technology, doctors and nurses may seem to perform miracles in saving a premature baby. But man and science just can not do as well in aiding the development of your baby in the ICN as Mother Nature could have done in the womb. The premature child comes into the world ahead of Nature's nine-month schedule, and the result is that it will be behind in development for quite some time.

Even if you judge the development of your child from the date that he should have been born and not the actual premature birth date, you will find that the child will lag behind a full-term infant. The premature child will take longer to focus his eyes on an object, to smile, to raise his head, to roll over, to stack blocks, to learn to talk. As parents, you must accept this slower development as a fact of life. But also, as parents, it is wise to focus more on the progress made than it is to spend excessive time comparing your infant's progress with the progress of your friends' children.

86. Will my premature child catch up in mental and physical growth with children who were born full-term?

If the child did not suffer any serious or lasting damage as the result of being born prematurely, he will be slower in development, but he will eventually catch up. However, it will take time. First, don't be disappointed at his progress, or lack of it. A book like *The First Twelve Months of Life: Your Baby's Growth Month by Month* by Frank Caplan is an excellent book, but it is not for the parents of preemies. You may use the book as a guide to see where a normal, full-term baby should be in terms of development, but don't expect your baby to be as advanced, even if you compute your baby's development from the time he or she should have been born.

Head circumference, a measure of brain growth, will usually be the first to catch up. Next will be length. Overall weight will be the last aspect of growth to catch up. Most parents are concerned with their preemie's weight, but it is the most misleading indicator of physical development. Head and overall length are much more important indicators of development. Pediatricians often tell parents that their premature child will catch up mentally by about grades one or two (ages six to seven) and physically about the time of adolescence (ages eleven to fourteen).

Accept your child's rate of development, and don't be too concerned about his shortcomings and failures when compared to other children his same age. After all, one premature child learned to speak very late, and in school, he actually failed math. His name was Albert Einstein.

87. Will there always be differences between my premature baby and "normal" children?

In the first year, or even two years, there may be obvious differences. Later in children's lives there may be no obvious differences whatsoever between pre-term and full-term babies. In the first year of life, however, one month can make a difference in how babies look and act. For example, pre-term babies' visual responsiveness may be more sluggish and their heads more wobbly because their muscles are not as developed. In time, the pre-term babies' muscles mature, but, if parents compare them with development of full-term babies born around the same time, they may become unnecessarily worried and frustrated.

When pre-term babies reach their expected due date, their faces look more mature than the faces of full-term babies born at the same time. Some parents may find reassurance in their baby's mature face; others may be misled to expect their babies to behave more maturely than they are biologically capable of and become disappointed.

88. Will my premature child have language problems?

That all depends on what you mean by language problems. If you consider late development of speech a problem, the answer will have to be yes. The premature child will take longer to begin talking, to say words, to learn new words, and to put those words into sentences. Generally speaking, the premature child of normal mentality without organic injury will begin the normal development landmarks in speech and language by the time he is two years old.

If the premature child is going to have a significant motor handicap, parents will usually see it by age one. The child may be slow to turn over, he may have difficulty learning to crawl, and if he does crawl, he may be slow in learning to walk. However, remember that most normal babies don't walk until after they are a year old, and the "nine month walker" is the exception rather than the rule. If your child is not crawling well by a year, see your pediatrician for advice and counsel. Predicting what a child's overall performance is going to be is a little more difficult. There is some data to suggest that looking at a child's mental performance at age two is an indicator of future performance. However, to judge all children's futures on age two performance is risky at best.

One of the things parents should look for is delays in language development. By age two, does the child have a vocabulary of twenty-five to fifty words? Does he respond to simple commands and directions, and indicate he knows more words than he can say? Does he show an interest in TV, especially the commercials? Does he like to be read to? If the answers to these questions are "no," there is obviously a delay in language development. Such a delay may indicate a problem with sensory input, such as seeing or hearing. However, it may also indicate mental retardation. Again, it will be one of those things you as a parent will begin wondering and worrying about when your child is two to three years old. If you suspect a language development problem, see your pediatrician for advice. As for language learning disabilities, it is not likely, even though the incidence of such disabilities is greater in premature children. Also, more boys than girls have language and reading disabilities, for reasons not yet known. Research shows that by the beginning of the past decade, between 80 and 90 percent of those "high risk" babies born at the nation's best prenatal centers did not suffer from any serious mental or physical problems. However, a more recent study has found that up to 48 percent of low birth weight children enter school with a major handicap, learning disability, or reading problem.

But it might be wise to put things in perspective. A few full-term children can read at three and a half to four years of age. Most can read easily at five to six years of age. A few are not ready for reading until age nine or ten. And some never acquire functional reading skill. Children in primary grades may be considered retarded readers or slow readers if they are six to twelve months behind grade placement. Keeping these facts in mind, you can make an adequate allowance for the slower development of your premature child. When your child begins reading, remember the attitudes of his peers and family members can exert profound influences on his motivation and acceptance of the written language. If you are a reader, and if you read to him, he will emulate you and be provided a role model that will encourage his reading. Also consider that his general motivation and interest in the content of the material to be read are powerful factors in his reading achievement. A wise parent will provide reading material of a high interest level when the child is ready for it.

89. Is there anything I can do to help my child's development?

This is a good question that has a positive answer. Yes, there are lots of things you can do to help your premature child catch up. First, your being aware that he will have a problem will help. Your acceptance of his slower rate of development will also help.

As for other things that you can do, I would suggest that you not talk "baby talk" around the child. Small babies, and especially premature babies because they are small so much longer, bring out all sorts of verbal gibberish from otherwise normal and articulate adults. It is difficult enough to learn a foreign language (which is what every baby must do) without having to learn something and then unlearn it later. Talk to your child in normal, standard English, but remember to keep it simple. When your child begins to learn words, make an extra effort to teach him the names of things. Words are the building blocks of human thinking and the more things he knows, the more he will be able to relate them to his experience and development. Teach him the names of objects in his environment— shoes, socks, chairs, toys, and so on. Let him experience abstract concepts like hot, cold, wet, or sharp by having him feel a warm cup of coffee, pick up an ice cube, splash in a water fountain, or experience the gentle prick of a safety pin. As he experiences the sensations, say the word.

As he learns nouns, repeat the names of those things when he sees them again or in different forms—on walks, in stores, or on TV. Watch TV with the child and name objects or animals as he sees them, especially during commercials. Flip through magazines or catalogues and name objects he knows and pick out new ones. As he progresses, play "I see" with him: "I see a red ball. Do you see a red ball?" This activity and repetition increases the child's knowledge of and mastery over his environment and increases his ability to learn new things.

Read to your child. Any child should be read to so that his language and imagination may develop, but a premature child especially needs to be read to. Reading will expose the child to new words and new ideas, and it will increase his curiosity and desire to learn to read for himself when he is able. And since everything we learn in life comes from experience, either firsthand experience or vicarious (secondhand) experience, reading will cause your child to experience many things in life that his immediate environment will not be able to provide firsthand.

Something else that you may be able to do that will help speech development is to teach your child nursery rhymes, short poems, or tongue twisters that will give him practice making sounds and manipulating words. Also, the abundance of children's stories and songs on records can be an aid, and they could prove to be a passive teacher while you are busy or away from your child.

A book that parents may find helpful is Stephen Lehane's *Help Your Baby Learn* (Prentice-Hall, 1976). It includes 100 Piaget-based activities for the first two years, and it shows parents how to use them to help their children learn important skills and sensory information at their own pace. But remember that the book is for full-term babies, and you must compensate for your child's lack of development. One other book parents may find helpful is *How to Raise a Brighter Child: The Case for Early Learning* by Joan Beck (Pocket Books, 1975). This book, by the respected writer of a syndicated column on child care, explains her theory on teaching and learning. It provides simple materials, games, and information that will make your preemie's first and most important teacher more effective.

Another thing that you can do is to be aware of your child's level of development in comparison to other children. Your child may not be ready for the experience of school at age six. His mental, emotional, and even physical development may be just far enough behind so that the experience of failure in school could do more damage than it is worth. You may be wise in planning to keep your child out of school a year if his lack of development warrants it. You may want to confer with your nursery school teacher or kindergarten teacher for suggestions, and an outside, objective opinion as to whether your child should delay starting school.

A FALECIA POSTSCRIPT

For those of you who may wonder about the loose ends in Falecia's story, I might add a few things. Of course there are always going to be loose ends and questions. After all, you have read a slice of life, not a neatly plotted story in which they all live happily ever after.

Well, I can tell you that the detached retina reattached itself without surgery, which was an almost miraculous occurrence. Falecia is not blind, as happens in the case of some preemies. She does not have perfect eyesight, and never will, but her nearsightedness is no worse than what her parents already have, and probably was caused more by her heredity than prematurity. It can easily be corrected by glasses when she gets old enough.

Developmentally, it was almost ten months before Falecia could smile and laugh, and as parents we were worried. But at twenty months she could say a number of words, including "cookie," her favorite. And she was adding more to her vocabulary. More importantly, she seemed to understand many more words than she could say. However, in every premature birth there are problems that may not have immediate solutions, and questions that may not have immediate answers. Only time will answer some of those questions as we watch Falecia grow and develop. So, I'll end our story by asking the same question I asked at the beginning. "How does it end?" The answer is still, "Who knows? It is still being written."

GLOSSARY

The parents of a preemie have lots of information tossed at them by a variety of people and sources in a short time. This information may be difficult to comprehend in a pressure situation. Although the handbook defines and explains most of the terms below, this glossary gives a quick definition for terms that you may hear doctors and nurses use when they talk about your infant. They may or may not explain the terms. Frequently they don't. It is easy for a person to assume that because one knows something, others know it too. However, the terms need to be known by parents in the early hours and long days of their child's stay in an ICN.

Ambu'ed. To have oxygen forced into the lungs with a balloon-like device. The term comes from a brand name of the device. (See Bagging.)

Amniocentesis. The analysis of amniotic fluid, a small amount of which is obtained through a needle inserted through the mother's abdomen and into the amniotic sac.

Anemia. A condition that exists when there are not enough red blood cells in the blood.

Apnea. The stopping of breathing, usually temporary in a preemie.

Aspiration. To draw out mucus and foreign material from the lungs and windpipe, or stomach by suction.

Bagging. A procedure used to temporarily help a baby to breathe. A small rubber bag attached to a mask is put over the baby's nose and mouth and air is pumped through the mask by squeezing the rubber bag, which forces oxygen into the baby's lungs.

Bilirubin. A product of the breakdown of dead red blood cells that causes jaundice if accumulated in the body. Bilirubin is processed by the liver and excreted in bile into the bowel.

Blood gas test. A test done on a drop or two of blood to determine the oxygen, acidity, and carbon dioxide levels in a baby's blood. The test results indicate what adjustments must be made in the baby's respiratory care.

Bonding. The emotional attachment that develops between parents and a baby, especially between a mother and her baby.

Bradycardia. A condition that exists when a baby's heart rate is slower than the normal 100-140 beats per minute.

Bronchopulmonary dysplasia. Scarring and damage to the lungs, often caused by forcing premature lungs to function before they are fully matured.

Catheter. Any tube used for putting fluids into a body or removing them from a body.

CBC (Complete Blood Count). A blood test to check for anemia, as well as signs of infection.

Chest tube. A tube passed through the chest wall and between the ribs. It is connected to a suction system to treat pneumothorax, or air leaking out of the lungs.

Colostrum. The milk first produced by a woman after birth. It is especially rich in antibodies and can provide the baby with many of the immunities from disease that the mother has developed.

CPAP (Continuous Positive Airway Pressure). The application of pressure to keep the lungs expanded. The expansion of the lungs is accomplished by a piece of equipment attached to a tube placed in the mouth or nose.

Edema. A condition that exists when there is too much fluid in the body tissues.

Electrode. An adhesive disc containing a wire, which is placed on the baby's chest to measure signals from the heart. Electrodes also measure chest expansion.

Endotracheal (ET) tube. A plastic tube that passes through the mouth or nose into the windpipe. It is connected to a respirator.

Fontanel. The "soft spot" of the head that all babies, including preemies, are born with. It eventually hardens and closes over as the skull matures.

Full-term infant. A baby born whose gestation age is between thirty-eight and forty-two weeks.

Gavage feeding. The feeding of a baby through a small plastic tube inserted through the mouth or nose and into the stomach.

Gestational age. The age of a baby from the date of conception to the date of delivery. A full-term baby has a gestational age of 38 to 42 weeks.

Heel stick. A method of obtaining blood samples by pricking the baby's heel.

Hemoglobin. The part of the red blood cells that contains iron. Hemoglobin is necessary to carry oxygen from the lungs to all other parts of the body.

Hyaline membrane disease. See respiratory distress syndrome.

Hyperalimentation. The administration of nutrients into a vein. It is used with infants who cannot be fed milk or formula.

ICN (Intensive Care Nursery). A special nursery for very sick or premature infants.

Incubator. A glass- or plastic-enclosed bed in which temperature and humidity may be controlled.

Intracranial hemorrhage. The breaking of fragile blood vessels in the brain; a stroke in a preemie.

Intravenous (IV). The administering of fluids through a hollow needle into a vein; often a vein in the head is used for preemies.

Intubation. The insertion of an endotracheal tube through the nose or mouth into the trachea, or windpipe.

IPPB (Intermittent Positive Pressure Breathing). A method used to assist breathing by placing a mask over the baby's nose and mouth to increase air pressure to inflate the lungs, then releasing pressure to allow the lungs to exhale.

Isolette. A brand name of a type of incubator. Often, any incubator is called an Isolette.

Jaundice. A condition in which the skin turns yellow because of too much bilirubin in the blood.

Lanugo. The fine body hair that preemies are often born with.

Lumbar puncture. A spinal tap, during which a small amount of the fluid which surrounds the baby's brain and spinal cord is withdrawn from the lower back for lab analysis.

Meconium. The dark, greenish material, composed of old swallowed blood, hair, and skin cells, found in a baby's intestines at birth.

Mucus. The fluid secreted by the membranes of the nose and throat.

Neonate. Any newborn baby.

Neonatologist. A physician specializing in the care of neonates, especially sick or premature newborns.

Open radiant warmer. An open crib with an overhead warmer to keep the preemie warm. It is usually used for babies that require extensive care, and it is easier for several people to work with such a baby than if it were in an incubator.

Oxyhood. A plastic shell that fits over the baby's head to provide oxygen and humidity.

Patent ductus arteriosis. The blood vessel that closes at birth in newborns, routing blood for the first time through the lungs to be oxygenated. In preemies, the vessel frequently does not close completely and must be closed by surgery and/or drug treatment.

Pediatrician. A doctor that specializes in the care of children.

Percussion. The procedure of tapping on a baby's chest to help the drainage of mucus, or to stimulate the heart in cases of bradycardia.

Phototherapy. The use of special fluorescent lights over a radiant warmer or Isolette in order to break down bilirubin; a treatment for jaundice.

Pneumothorax. A condition in which air leaks from the baby's lungs into the chest cavity surrounding the lung, causing it to collapse.

Premature infant. One born before thirty-eight weeks of gestational age.

Respirator. A machine that breathes for the baby.

Respiratory distress syndrome (RDS). A respiratory disorder in which there is a tendency for the air sacs of the lungs to collapse. It is often seen in preemies and is usually due to underdevelopment.

Retrolental fibroplasia. A condition in preemies that results in increased fragility and growth of blood vessels in and around the retina. The blood vessel growth and breakage cause damage to the immature retina and can seriously damage sight. Although associated with premature infants requiring oxygen, its exact cause remains the subject of extensive research.

Sepsis. An overwhelming infection in the blood or tissues of the body.

Tachycardia. Rapid heart rate, greater than 150 beats per minute.

TPN (Total Parenteral Nutrition). A formula that is given the infant by an IV.

Trachea. The windpipe.

Transpyloric feeding. A method of feeding either breast milk or formula through a small tube passed through the stomach and into the small intestine.

Umbilical artery catheter. A plastic tube placed in one of the arteries of the umbilical cord so that fluids can be infused into the body or blood drawn from the body. The umbilicus normally has two arteries and one vein.

Urinalysis. A laboratory examination of the urine.

Now that you have finished this book, the authors would like some advice and opinions. Because each premature baby is an individual and each is a special case, it is impossible to cover everything that may be of importance and concern to you, despite the fact that the experience of thousands of parents went into this book's preparation. So, your comments and suggestions would be greatly appreciated.

_____ Did you find this book helpful?
_____ Did you find this book informative?
_____ Did you find this book comforting?
_____ Did it cover all your problems and questions?
_____ Yes _____ No _____ To Some Extent

If not, what other concerns need to be addressed? (List them below.)

Please tear out this page and mail to:

Dr. Bernard Griesemer
Sunshine Pediatrics, Inc.
3014 "J" East Sunshine
Springfield, MO 65804

INDEX

In the index below the boldface numbers refer to the numbers of the questions under which an answer containing the desired information appears. The numbers not in boldface type refer to pages of the personal narrative, which deal with one family's experiences and reactions to that topic or subject.

If you found this book to be valuable and informative and you know a parent, doctor, nurse, or social worker who would also find it helpful, please note the information below. Because a premature birth is usually unexpected, a parent is more than likely not to have information dealing with the problems.

In addition, many smaller bookstores stock only books which sell fast and frequently, and they may not carry a "specialized" book like this. You may be doing someone a good turn by ordering it for him or her directly or by passing on the information so that such people in need may order it themselves.

Please send me the following copy(s) of *The Littlest Baby* (Pfister & Griesemer) as specified below:

_____ Hardcover @ $12.95 (537795-1) $_____

_____ Paperback @ $5.95 (537787-0) $_____

Please add 50¢ per book for postage and handling. $_____

☐ Yes, please send me the Spectrum Catalogue
of all your fine books (50¢) $_____

                                    Total $_____

Enclosed is my ☐ check   ☐ money order
or charge my   ☐ Visa   ☐ MasterCard

Account # _____ Expiration date_____

Name_____

Address_____

City_____

Cut out and mail this form to Prentice-Hall, Inc.
                    Att: Addison Tredd
                    General Publishing Division
                    Englewood Cliffs, NJ 07632

Prices subject to change without notice. Please allow 4 weeks for delivery.